THE MAUDSLEY
Maudsley Monographs

MAUDSLEY MONOGRAPHS

HENRY MAUDSLEY, from whom the series of monographs takes its name, was the founder of The Maudsley Hospital and the most prominent English psychiatrist of his generation. The Maudsley Hospital was united with the Bethlem Royal Hospital in 1948 and its medical school, renamed the Institute of Psychiatry at the same time, became a constituent part of the British Postgraduate Medical Federation. It is now associated with King's College, London, and entrusted with the duty of advancing psychiatry by teaching and research. The Bethlem-Maudsley NHS Trust, together with the Institute of Psychiatry, are jointly known as The Maudsley.

The monograph series reports work carried out at The Maudsley. Some of the monographs are directly concerned with clinical problems; others, less obviously relevant, are in scientific fields that are cultivated for the furtherance of psychiatry.

Maudsley Monographs number forty-three

Developing a national mental health policy

Rachel Jenkins
*Visiting Professor and Director of the WHO Collaborating Centre
Institute of Psychiatry, London, UK
Visiting Professor, London School of Hygiene and Tropical Medicine
Visiting Scholar, Green College, Oxford*

Andrew McCulloch
The Sainsbury Centre for Mental Health, London, UK

Lynne Friedli
Mentality, UK

Camilla Parker
*Consultant in mental health law and policy
Non-executive Director of Camden and Islington Mental Health
NHS Trust
Consultant to the Mental Disability Advocacy Program, Open Science
Institute, Budapest*

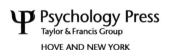
Ψ Psychology Press
Taylor & Francis Group

HOVE AND NEW YORK

Published 2014 by Psychology Press
27 Church Road, Hove, East Sussex, BN3 2FA, UK
711 Third Avenue, New York, NY 10017

First issued in paperback 2015

Psychology Press is an imprint of the Taylor and Francis Group, an informa business

First received: May 2000
Final revision: February 2001
Pre-publication copy requested by Editor-in-chief, World Health Report, March 2001

British Library Cataloguing in Publication Data
A catalogue record for this book is available from the British Library

Library of Congress Cataloging in Publication Data
Developing a national mental health policy / Rachel Jenkins ... [et al.].
    p. cm. — (Maudsley monographs ; no. 43)
   Includes bibliographical references and index.
   ISBN 1-84169-295-6
   1. Mental health policy—United States. 2. Mental health planning—United States. I.
Jenkins, Rachel. II. Series.

 RA790.6 .D48 2002
 362.2'0973—dc21

                                                                                2001048476
ISBN13: 978-1-138-87195-3 (pbk)
ISBN13: 978-1-84169-295-1 (hbk)

ISSN 0076-5465

Typeset by Quorum Technical Services Ltd, Cheltenham

Contents

Acknowledgements

We gratefully acknowledge contributions from Dr Gyles Glover (the main author of the section on mental health information systems); Dr Geraldine Strathdee, who contributed to the section on primary care; Dr Florence Muja and Betty Bigombe, who both contributed to the section on trauma; and Mary Hancock, who wrote the section on the contribution of religious groups and churches to the care and support of people with mental illness. Rebecca Bazeley, a voluntary researcher working for Dr McCulloch, helped to develop the typology of the different cultural and historical views of mental health problems. We are very grateful to Derek Flannery for his work checking and collating references.

Foreword 1

Mental illness causes a substantial health burden in all regions of the world. This burden is not only from disability and suicide, but also from the loss of economic productivity, family burden, reduced access to and success of health promotion, prevention and treatment programmes, and mortality from the associated vulnerability to physical disease, including infectious diseases.

The goal of DFID is the alleviation of poverty. Mental health differentially affects the poor and impedes the achievement of other health and development targets. Therefore DFID welcomes the timely publication of this important book which is designed to support those involved in developing locally appropriate mental health policies in the different regions of the world, and to increase local capacity in policy, strategic development and implementation.

The book takes a broad and contextual approach to mental health policy, emphasising the crucial role of primary care, NGOs, the social sector, schools and workplaces, and the criminal justice system as well as the specialist services. It highlights the importance of liaison at national, regional and local levels between the relevant sectors, and contains very useful chapters on the principles of human rights and mental health legislation, mental health information systems and human resource strategies. The important issues of accountability and financing are considered, as well as key cultural issues and the importance of dialogue with traditional healers. The book represents an excellent, practical and supportive guide for those who should be engaged in mental health, and will be an invaluable tool as we work towards promoting, protecting and improving mental health in poor countries, and the incorporation of mental health issues into broader health sector and poverty reduction processes.

Julian Lob Levyt
Department for International Development (DFID), UK

Foreword 2

This book is a major achievement, and fulfils an important need in many countries of the world. All nations need a mental health policy, but few people have the detailed knowledge to produce one, and most have no idea how to set about the task. It is a 'how to do it' book: it gives detailed information on what to collect beforehand, then gives guidance for each step of the way. It also lists those sections of the community that should be involved – government departments, the pharmaceutical and insurance industries, voluntary agencies, religious organisations and user and carer groups – and provides valuable advice on inter-agency working and mental health promotion.

The book is strikingly comprehensive, and is written with knowledge of the public health impact of mental disorder on the people of the world. Rightly there is major emphasis on the needs to strengthen the mental health aspects of primary care, but the authors do not lose sight of the fact that specialist mental health services are also a vital part of overall services.

The authors wisely refrain from attempting to impose Western views on developing countries. They have comprehensive and up-to-date knowledge of services in many parts of the developing world, linked with great admiration for the work of pioneering colleagues in those countries who have adapted the pattern of mental health services to the needs of developing countries in the post-institutional era. They are aware that mental health services need to be adapted to take account not only of the cultures in individual countries, but also of different levels of available resources, different natural resources and different climates.

Where human rights are concerned, they list the 18 points of the principles relevant to the mentally ill, as well as providing reminders of the Universal Declaration on Human Rights, and the International Covenant on civil and political rights.

Although the authors describe many innovative mental health systems, throughout the world much remains to be done. There are still many patients incarcerated in large institutions, and a substantial proportion of the rural populations of the developing world still have no mental health services whatever. A major task in many countries is to train a new cadre of mental health workers, who may be trained mental nurses, multi-purpose health workers, or even volunteers such as the Lady Health Workers beginning to be set up in rural Pakistan.

Progress is impossible without some central determination to change: this book provides the guidance and points the way forward.

David Goldberg
Professor Emeritus
Institute of Psychiatry, King's College
London

How to use this book

This book is aimed at all those seeking to develop a national or strategic mental health policy. It is particularly aimed at

- Government officials
- Politicians
- Officials in national agencies with an interest in mental health
- Clinicians and professionals seeking to influence policy
- Staff in NGOs seeking to influence policy
- Staff in unions, trade organisations and other agencies with an interest in mental health.

However, within this target audience different individuals will be starting at different points in terms of their knowledge of mental health and/or government and strategic planning mechanisms. Some users of the book will wish to read it through from beginning to end, while others may wish to refer only to specific sections. Those with a core interest in strategic planning of mental health services may wish to concentrate on Chapters 1–7. More specifically, the following signposts for each chapter may be helpful:

Chapter 1: *Introductory issues* – of general interest, but of lesser importance to those who are highly familiar with concepts of mental health and mental illness.

Chapter 2: *Public health burden* – of fundamental importance to those wishing to make the case for a national mental health strategy.

Chapter 3: *The strategy* – the heart of the book, detailing the key elements of a mental health strategy.

Chapter 4: *Legislation* – of particular relevance to those seeking to introduce or amend mental health legislation.

Chapter 5: *Mental health information systems* – related to Chapter 11. This chapter discusses an infrastructure issue relevant to implementation.

Chapter 6: *Mental health promotion* – also fundamental. Mental health promotion is the neglected arm of national and world strategies to improve mental health.

Chapter 7: *Primary care* – again, this is likely to be relevant to almost all readers. Tackling mental health problems in primary care in an appropriate way is essential.

Chapter 8: *Specialist care and links to primary care* – will probably be relevant to most readers.

Chapter 9: *Inter-agency working* – also relevant to most readers, but of particular concern in countries with complex organisational structures.

Chapter 10: *Tackling mortality* – relevant to all. This chapter addresses the links between physical and mental health.

Chapter 11: *Investing for the future* – deals with the long-term investment strategies required as part of an overall mental health plan.

Chapter 12: *Some special priorities* – deals with subgroups of the population which might require special attention.

Chapter 13 and 14: *Traditional healers and disasters* – of particular relevance to some countries with large numbers of traditional healers, or to countries that have suffered recent disasters.

Chapter 15: *Common problems* – usefully read by all those seeking to develop a strategy sensitive to local problems and weaknesses.

Glossary

Most terms and concepts used in this book are defined in the accompanying text. However, a few terms are used without accompanying definitions and those are given here. (The definitions with an asterisk have been adapted from Davies, 2000.)

Assertive outreach*   A system of intensive client centered community support, including health care and social support, for people with severe mental illness who have difficulty in engaging with services. It is characterized by low caseloads and a high regular and persistent contact with clients.

Care   Health and social care by both formal and informal carers.

Carers   People who informally care for someone with mental illness, e.g. family, neighbours and friends.

Care planning*   This consists of needs assessment (see below), followed by the formulation of an agreed plan as to how those needs are to be met. The plan is usually developed in a multidisciplinary way, involving the relevant professionals, patient and carer. The concept has evolved in specialist care but could also be used in primary care.

Case management*   This term refers to a patient-centred system of care, with a strong emphasis on the co-ordination of care in the community. Its goals are continuity of care and individualised support through assessment, care planning, intervention, monitoring and review. There are many models of case management.

Commissioner   Someone, often an administrator or public health doctor at district level, who requests a specific service infrastructure from a health provider.

Community alliances   Partnerships or joint working between formal and informal community organisations.

Evidence-based medicine   The practice of medicine in accordance with the best available research evidence.

Mental health   Includes a positive sense of well-being; individual resources including self-esteem, optimism, a sense of mastery and coherence; the ability to initiate, develop and sustain mutually satisfying personal relationships and the ability to cope with adversities.

Mental health problems   Include psychological distress usually connected with various life situations, events and problems; common mental disorders (e.g. depression, anxiety disorders); severe mental disorders with disturbances in perception, beliefs and thought processes (psychoses); substance abuse disorders (excess consumption and dependency on alcohol, drugs, tobacco); abnormal personality traits which are handicapping to the individual and/or to others; and progressive organic disorders of the brain (dementias).

Mental health promotion   An interdisciplinary and socio-cultural endeavour geared to enhancing the well-being of individuals, groups and communities. It implies the creation of individual, social, societal and environmental conditions which enable optimal psychological development and reduction in mental health problems.

Needs assessment*   Individual assessment of the range of physical, psychological and social needs of a service user or patient. It should cover both the range of needs that can be met by services and also needs that are not necessarily able to be met within current knowledge or resources. It is the first step in the care planning process.

NGO   Non-governmental organisation.

Primary care   The first point of contact with the patient, user or client, providing non-specialised care and an overview of health and social care needs. Primary care is sometimes provided by specialist services working in a more generalist mode (e.g. A&E departments, assertive outreach teams) but it is usually provided by general practitioners and primary care nurses.

Risk assessment   Prediction of likelihood that an individual will commit violence directed to self and others.

Stakeholder   Someone with a specific and legitimate interest in mental health services who should therefore be consulted.

User   A consumer of services, client, patient. It is *not* used in this book in the sense of someone who uses illicit drugs.

User advocacy   Independent advocacy or support for users of mental health services, usually from other users or trained lay volunteers, to enable them to make their voices heard with statutory and non-statutory agencies.

User involvement   Users being involved in actual delivery of services, in decision-making about service policy and planning, and in training activities.

Table acknowledgements

We are grateful for permission from the Editor, British Journal of Psychiatry, to reproduce Tables 10.2, 10.3, and 10.4, which originally appeared in Volume 173, pp. 11–53, Harris, E.C. and Barraclough, B. *Excess mortality of mental disorder*.

CHAPTER ONE

Introductory issues:
Mental health and mental illness

Key Points

- *Mental health is of fundamental strategic importance.*
- *The economic and social burden of mental ill health is massive, and mental illness contributes to poverty.*
- *Poor mental health impacts on physical health.*
- *Mental ill health needs to be addressed at all life stages, and at all levels of society in a range of settings.*
- *There are different models of mental ill health world wide which need to be understood and respected.*

MENTAL HEALTH: ITS VALUE, RELEVANCE AND STRATEGIC IMPORTANCE

Action on mental health across the world is of fundamental strategic importance because of the contribution of mental health and the impact of mental illness on social, human and economic capital. Therefore, this book seeks to give theoretical and practical support to governmental and non-governmental agencies wishing to develop and improve mental health policy and implementation.

The book addresses both the promotion of good mental health and effective interventions for specific mental illness, both severe and milder conditions. There is no conflict here. Unless the whole system of mental health care is managed appropriately it will not function effectively. It is right that more specialised services focus on those with severe problems, as well as providing support to generic services to address more common problems. A crucial aspect of mental health policy is to get this balance right – and there will clearly be legitimate variations in the exact balance from society to society. Decisions on the precise balance to be struck will depend on a variety of factors including the views of stakeholders, in particular service users and mental health professionals.

The strategic importance of mental ill health

Mental ill health is not simply an absence of good mental health. While some individuals undoubtedly suffer from a generalised sense of poor mental well-being, there are specific forms of mental illness that have huge and well-recognised impacts on individuals, families and societies. These crucially include depression, schizophrenia and manic-depressive illness.

If these illnesses are not managed in an optimal way by health and social care systems, there are a number of major negative consequences:

- Primary care services can be overwhelmed with minor or moderate psychiatric problems, sometimes presenting as chronic physical health problems.
- Those with more severe illnesses may not be treated in the appropriate part of the system, leading to poorer functioning and more frequent breakdowns.
- There are major social consequences in terms of disrupted working life, dysfunctional families, disrupted education and, of course, individual suffering.
- Mental illness contributes to individual and national poverty (for example: lost production from people being unable to work; reduced productivity from people who are ill at work; lost production from absenteeism; accidents at work; lost production from premature death; loss of the breadwinner of a dependent family; unwanted pregnancy; untreated childhood disorders leading to educational failure, hence to unemployment and to illness in adult life; untreated parental disorders leading to childhood disorders and a cycle of disadvantage).

In addressing severe mental health problems, it is important to take a broad view to the needs of individual patients or service users. This will mean that the strategy for addressing severe mental health problems must look at the broad spectrum of patient needs – including welfare, social integration, housing and daily occupation as well as health care.

The value of mental health

Mental health is more than an absence of symptoms of mental illness or distress. Mental health refers to a positive sense of well-being and a belief in our own worth and the dignity and worth of others (HEA, 1998a).

Positive mental health includes the capacity to perceive, comprehend and interpret our surroundings, to adapt to them and to change them if necessary, to think and speak coherently, and to communicate with each other. Mental health also affects our ability to cope with and manage change, transition and life events: the birth of a child, unemployment, bereavement or physical ill-health. Thus mental health is an essential component of general health (Lavaikainen et al., 2001).

Mental health is mediated by the quality of interaction with others, societal structures and resources, and cultural values. Socio-economic factors – notably education, employment, income distribution and housing – play an important role.

Mental health and well-being are issues of everyday life and should be of interest to every citizen and employer, in addition to all care, education and administration sectors. Mental health is influenced (enhanced or jeopardised) in families and schools, on the streets and in workplaces – where people can feel safe, respected, included and able to participate or may be in fear, marginalised or excluded. It is the result of, among other things, the way we are treated by others, and the way we treat other people and ourselves. Everyone has mental health needs, whether or not they have a diagnosis of mental illness. Mental health promotion is therefore relevant to everyone.

The importance of mental health promotion

The case for investment in mental health promotion extends far beyond its impact on the prevalence of mental illness, e.g. depression, anxiety or schizophrenia. The consequences of poor mental health can be seen in a wide range of health, social and economic problems. One of the reasons for the low level of investment in mental health promotion is the global failure to make the links between mental well-being and social functioning and productivity.

In many countries, policy initiatives and strategies for mental health are in reality concerned almost exclusively with the treatment and prevention of mental illness. Psychological variables (e.g. levels of self-esteem) and life skills (e.g. communication, negotiation and conflict management) – 'protective factors' – have a significant mediating influence on the impact of socio-economic factors on health, and individual, family or community responses to trauma or stressful life events. The impact of risk factors for mental health problems, for example, bereavement, or a family history of psychiatric disorder or unemployment, can be reduced by strengthening factors known to protect mental well-being. Many risk factors for mental health problems are, however, difficult to address, notably those arising from political conflicts, long-term economic problems or natural disasters.

A strategic framework for mental health promotion therefore needs to achieve a balance between reducing risk factors and strengthening protective factors which can enhance the ability of communities to cope with and survive difficulties.

HOW DO DIFFERENT CULTURES VIEW MENTAL HEALTH PROBLEMS?

There has been debate for centuries, within a variety of cultures, about what is meant by 'mental health problems'. Mental disorder was identified in most or all cultures as far back as we have detailed written records. The early Greek philosophers and doctors wrote about it in some detail using biological, psychological and spiritual explanations (see, for example, Jones, 1972). The Bible, the Koran, and other holy books refer to different kinds of mental disorder, sometimes in terms of demon possession or other spiritual disturbances, but the 'symptoms' are referred to in recognisable ways (e.g. the descriptions of what are now called epilepsy and schizo-phrenia in the Christian Gospels). The first recorded mental health institution was founded in Damascus in the eighth century AD and functioned according to Islamic principles. Clearly, an understanding of the needs of mentally ill people long predates modern psychiatry.

Explanations of mental health problems remain varied today. Different religions, cultural groups and professions adopt different models of the causes of mental illness, while essentially talking about the same under-lying phenomena. These different explanations and terminology need to be recognised and respected. The objective of introducing modern mental health services is to meet people's needs and improve their health and social functioning, not to influence them to adhere to a particular world view or ideology. It is better to work *with* the grain of local or regional explanations of mental disorder than *against* it.

Broadly speaking, views of mental illness can be divided into the four main groups detailed below.

- *Biological*. This includes the so-called 'medical model' of a physically (neurological or biochemical) based disease including genetic, endocrine, nutritional and traumatic explanations. Such explanations are offered by some doctors although most psychiatrists will integrate the biological aspects of an illness, if present, with the social and psychological aspects. Biological explanations may also be used by the general public.

- *Social/psychological*. This is the second strand of scientific thinking used by psychologists and other professionals as well as many psychia-trists. It uses a conceptual aetiological framework of life events, social stresses, social support and psychological mechanisms such as coping mechanisms and locus of control. It is relevant to all mental illnesses, contributing to symptoms and functioning, but is particularly relevant to depression and anxiety. Again, this view has some standing with lay audiences and is also attractive to many patients/service users.

- *Intuitive/spiritual*. These are models which use creative explanations of mental phenomena and depict the mind as battlegrounds for opposing forces. They range through psychoanalytic models to spirit possession. Spirit possession remains a common explanation for severe mental illness in many cultures within developed societies and should not be associated only with cultures in low-income countries. It should not be assumed that such models are always unhelpful (e.g. Neki et al., 1986; Beneduce, 1996) or that the interventions associated with them are always ineffective (e.g. Englund, 1998). For an analysis of Jewish and Christian responses to mental health problems see *Mental Health Promotion: The Role of Faith Communities – Jewish and Christian Perspectives* (HEA, 1999b).

- *Existential*. This model is rarer, viewing mental 'disorder' as just another valid form of human existence. It is present in some Eastern cultures and also in parts of the Western user movement.

The distinction between the biological and the social models is increasingly blurred as scientific research demonstrates that even in severe psychosis, where there is usually some genetic contribution, social and psychological factors remain important in both aetiology and outcome. Likewise in mild–moderate depression and anxiety, hitherto thought to be completely environmentally determined, there is now evidence of a genetic contribution in some cases. Most psychiatrists and other mental health professionals acknowledge and integrate the relevance of all these concepts into a multidimensional assessment and management framework for their patients which addresses physical, social and psychological needs.

Mental illness is not synonymous with social deviancy

Several distinguished psychiatrists and lawyers have warned strongly against defining mental illness in terms of socially deviant behaviour (Lewis 1953; Wootton 1959). The United Nations' *Principles for the Protection of Persons with Mental Illness* (discussed in more detail in Chapter 4) state that:

> 'A determination of mental illness shall never be made on the basis of political, economic or social status, or membership in a cultural, racial or religious group, or for any other reason not directly relevant to mental health status.' (Principle 4(2))

If mental illness is inferred from socially deviant behaviour alone political abuse may result. Mental illness undoubtedly has social causes and social consequences, but it is defined by the presence of a disturbance in psychological functions such as perception, memory, emotion, learning, thinking, etc., and not by abnormal social behaviour which may or may not be additionally present.

IMPLICATIONS OF DIFFERENT VIEWS OF MENTAL ILLNESS FOR THE OVERALL STRATEGY

The need to take account of the differing views of mental illness

It is important to have some understanding of the different views of mental illness, which may exist in any country or society, in order to tackle practical issues around communicating with stakeholders and deciding on and presenting a strategy for a particular country or setting. We learn from our own culture and ethnic backgrounds how to be ill. The meanings attached to the notions of health and illness are related to basic culture-bound values by which we define a given experience and perception (Spector, 1979). Therefore it is important to know the cultural background of the people and their conceptions of diseases and illnesses.

While qualified professionals world wide will increasingly tend to hold multiaxial biological/social/psychological views of mental illness, which are almost always also the basis of mental health legislation world wide, the general population and other important stakeholders – such as spiritual leaders, elders and health care workers, who are not formally qualified – may not. Those experiencing mental health problems and their families and friends who care for them (carers), will also have viewpoints that need to be taken into account and respected.

In addition to understanding the different views within the relevant country or setting, the following points should be borne in mind:

- While the scientific evidence favours the bio-psychosocial model, stakeholder views should be respected and taken into consideration in strategy formulation.
- Sometimes a specific explanatory model of mental illness (e.g. spirit possession) may lead to unhelpful or even harmful interventions. This will need to be planned for and considered. It may not always be necessary to confront such models head on. It may be helpful to encourage the distinction between mental health problems and moral and spiritual manifestations of evil which require disapproval.

- Models of mental illness will be deeply embedded in the various stakeholder groups as they stem from experience, observation and training. One way forward in developing a joint strategy is sometimes to get the stakeholders to agree on the priority needs of mentally ill people and what opportunities they need to be offered, rather than on precisely what they suffer from.
- As well as understanding how the local community population views mental illness, it is important to understand how it is viewed by the traditional healers, the concepts they hold, and how they treat it. Sometimes the herbal medicines used are pharmacologically active. Sometimes rituals of spirit exorcism involve the family and neighbours in a way that can beneficially alter the family dynamics, which may have been a source of considerable stress to the patient.

Service strategies need to take account of local understanding of mental illness and of traditional methods of healing, and mental health professionals need to understand and take account of the individual patient's understanding of his or her illness, and its causes. It is also possible that the meaning of being psychologically ill and seeking treatment for one's psychiatric condition may have different connotations and impact in various cultures, which in turn may influence the course of a disorder and its outcome – and this may be a partial explanation for the more favourable outcome of schizophrenia in low-income countries (Jablensky et al., 1992; Kulhara, 1994; *see also* Institute of Medicine, 2001).

The value of classification and the dangers of labelling

Classification of mental disorders has always been more contentious than classification of physical illness. This is partly because, with a few exceptions, psychiatric diagnoses tend to be based entirely on the clinical features of the illness rather than on a pathological test; partly because the therapeutic and prognostic implications of psychiatric diagnoses are relatively weak until combined with information on severity and disability; and partly because there is undoubted evidence that attaching diagnostic labels may be stigmatising and socially harmful (Goffman, 1961; Bhugra & Buchanan, 1993).

Inevitably, therefore, terminology of mental disorders is controversial. Much of the Western mental health user movement resists the use of psychiatric terminology which it regards as unhelpful and damaging labelling, and it is important to recognise the validity of this message, whether we agree with it or not. There is plenty of evidence that psychiatric labels may be damaging and modify society's behaviour to the labelled individual in an unhelpful and sometimes catastrophic way.

There is a significant difference between the overall process of classification – which seeks to group related disorders in order to understand them, treat them or respond effectively – and the individual result of being labelled which identifies the person with the disorder and embodies potentially inaccurate assumptions about that person's capabilities and behaviour. Stigma means that there is a tendency in most societies to move from clinically useful diagnosis to unhelpful social labelling. This is why both anti-stigma campaigns and mental health promotion (in its sense of promoting the value which society places on mental health as well as the overall promotion of mental health of a population) are fundamental to a mental health strategy.

In view of these shortcomings, why does classification persist? The reason is that only by classifying illness can therapeutic knowledge increase. The essence of a diagnosis is that it embodies as many as possible of those characteristics that are common to several different patients, and not only allows research studies to be done on the prevalence of disorders and the effectiveness of treatments, but also allows communication about patients and knowledge of efficacious treatments to be disseminated.

However, for clinical purposes, the need for a classification system and operational diagnoses does not militate against the need for a formulation of every person with a mental disorder, which aims to appreciate and understand the unique features of that person, his or her environment, and the interaction between them. Such a formulation is essential for any real understanding of the person and planning his or her overall care, but is unusable in any situation in which whole populations or groups of patients need to be considered (Johnstone, 1998).

International classifications

International classifications of mental disorders have existed for over a century, and have become widely used in most countries in the last 30 years. There are two main international classification systems in current use: the International Classification of Diseases, Injuries and Causes of Death (8th revision 1969, 9th revision 1979) and the 10th revision is now known as the *International Statistical Classification of Diseases and Related Health Problems*, referred to as ICD-10). The other is the American Psychiatric Association's *Diagnostic and Statistical Manual of Mental Disorders*, first published in 1952, and now on its 4th revision (referred to as DSM-IV).

ICD-10 is a single axis classification but DSM-IV (like its predecessors) advocates the use of five axes to promote consideration of all relevant aspects of clinical situations. The criteria developed in international classifications to delineate the categories and severity of mental disorders are made use of in survey methodology (see below).

Using classification categories to plan policy and services

For the purposes of planning mental health policy and services, there is a key group of broad categories of illness that need to be considered, but the fine detail of the international classifications and their differences is not very important in this context. The broad categories that have been found to be helpful for planning purposes comprise:

- depression
- anxiety
- emotional and conduct disorder in children
- schizophrenia
- bipolar affective disorder
- dementia
- substance abuse
- eating disorders
- antisocial personality disorder, and
- intellectual disability (learning disability).

All these categories of disorder, apart from eating disorders, are ubiquitous, and found in every country in the world. Eating disorders were relatively unknown in low-income countries, although recent studies are demonstrating rising rates with increasing Westernisation (e.g. Lee, 1996; Lee & Lee, 2000).

Standardised research instruments – questionnaires and structured or semi-structured interviews – have been developed, tested and used widely round the world over the last few decades, allowing estimates of prevalence, incidence, outcome and examination of associated risk factors (e.g. Thompson, 1989). Whereas early studies in the 1950s and 1960s showed that the reliability of psychiatric diagnoses was often very low, the introduction of structured interviews and operational definitions has transformed the situation. There has been considerable attention to, and investigation of, the transcultural performance of several instruments, e.g. Goldberg et al. (1997) who found that the widely used screening instrument, the General Health Questionnaire, performed just as well in detecting cases of depression and anxiety in low-income countries as in the Western world.

The broad categories of mental disorder

Depression and anxiety

These are the commonest conditions frequently occurring in a mixed form (mixed anxiety-depression) (Barbee, 1998). Depression is characterised by low mood, fatigue, irritability, poor concentration, impaired sleep, appetite and libido, low self-esteem and feelings of worthlessness. It may be accompanied by suicidal feelings. Symptoms of anxiety may be acutely episodic (panic disorder), including palpitations, sweating, trembling, feelings of unreality and a fear of dying. Such episodes may occur in specific situations (agoraphobia and specific phobias), or may be generalised (generalised anxiety disorder).

Epidemiological studies from all regions of the world have shown that these conditions are common in community populations (e.g. Kessler et al., 1994; Jenkins et al., 1998a; Parry, 1996), in people at work (Jenkins, 1985a) and in primary care populations (Ormel et al., 1994; Ustun & Sartorius, 1995). They contribute to sickness absence (Jenkins, 1985b) and labour turnover (Jenkins, 1985c) and form a significant contribution to the overall public health burden of mental disorder (Murray & Lopez, 1996). The epidemiology of depression and schizophrenia in populations across the world have recently been reviewed (Jenkins, 2001a; Jablensky, 2001).

Schizophrenia

This term covers a group of disorders characterised by fundamental and characteristic distortions of thinking and perception, including delusions and hallucinations (usually auditory). In the characteristic schizophrenic disturbance of thinking, peripheral and irrelevant features of a total concept are brought to the fore instead of those that are relevant and appropriate, so thinking becomes vague, elliptical and obscure, and speech may be incomprehensible. Mood is flattened or incongruous. The course of the disorder is very variable, with a proportion chronic and relapsing, a proportion deteriorating, and some attaining complete recovery.

Schizophrenia is found in all countries and cultures and has a life-time prevalence of between 7 and 9 per 1000 (Jablensky et al., 1986). The point prevalence varies between around 2 and 5 per 1000. Collaborative studies by the World Health Organisation have shown that the prevalence of schizophrenia, when assessed in comparable ways, is similar in different countries (Jablensky et al., 1992). Although much rarer than depression and anxiety, it too forms a significant contribution to the overall public health burden because of the chronicity, deterioration, and extreme social disability in a proportion of sufferers. The outcome of schizophrenia is probably more favourable in developing countries than in the West, but the reasons are not yet clear (Kulhara, 1994).

Bipolar affective disorder

This disorder is characterised by repeated episodes in which the person's mood and activity levels are significantly disturbed, sometimes with elevation of mood, increased energy and activity (mania or hypomania) and sometimes with lowered mood and decreased energy and activity (depression). Recovery is usually complete between episodes. Like schizophrenia, it is relatively rare, but important in public health terms because of the severity of the episodes and the need for relapse protection.

Dementia

Dementia covers a group of diseases of the brain, usually of a chronic or progressive nature, in which there is disturbance of memory, thinking, orientation, comprehension, calculation, learning capacity, language and judgement. Consciousness is not clouded, unlike in delirium. Cognitive impairment is accompanied by deterioration in emotional control, social behaviour, or motivation and ability to accomplish tasks of daily living. It occurs in Alzheimer's disease, in cerebrovascular disease and in other conditions such as infections, toxins, cancers and metabolic disorders affecting the brain.

The prevalence of moderate and severe dementia is about 5% of people aged 65 and over and 20% of those aged over 80 (Henderson, 1986). The total number of people with dementia is increasing rapidly as life expectancy improves and this is an important issue for established market economies, and an increasingly important issue for the developing countries where life expectancy is now also increasing rapidly.

Substance abuse

This refers to harmful use of psychoactive substances which may result in damage to health, dependence syndrome, and adverse social damage. Alcohol and drug abuse are both contributors to important social problems, and are often associated with psychiatric disorders such as depression, anxiety or schizophrenia.

The prevalence varies with social and cultural factors which influence availability and access to the psychoactive substances, and these will vary from country to country. For example, it is now widely accepted that the proportion of the population drinking excessively is closely related to the average consumption of that population (Ledermann, 1956; Smith, 1981).

Eating disorders

These disorders include syndromes of overeating (bulimia nervosa) and deliberate weight loss (anorexia nervosa). The prevalence may be 1–2% in schoolgirls and female university students in Western countries. It is rarely seen in non-Western countries or in the non-White population of Western countries (Szmuckler, 1985).

Antisocial personality disorder

Personality disorder is a severe disturbance of character and behavioural tendencies which appears in late childhood and continues through adult life. The abnormal behaviour pattern is enduring, or long standing and not limited to episodes of mental illness. The disorder is usually, but not invariably, associated with significant problems in social and occupational performance. There are several kinds of personality disorder, for example, anxious, schizoid, paranoid personality disorders, but the one that is most significant for planning purposes is antisocial personality disorder or psychopathic personality disorder. This is characterised by callous unconcern for the feelings of others; gross and persistent attitudes of irresponsibility and disregard for social norms, rules and obligation; incapacity to maintain enduring relationships although no difficulty establishing them; very low tolerance to frustration and a very low threshold for discharge of aggression including violence; and an incapacity to experience guilt or to profit from experience, particularly punishment. It may follow on from conduct disorder in childhood. Although there have been many studies of this disorder in prisons and secure psychiatric hospitals where it is common, very few data are available on its prevalence in community populations.

Learning disability

Learning disability, intellectual handicap or mental retardation is characterised by a reduced level of intellectual functioning which results in diminished ability to adapt to the daily demands of the normal social environment. The intelligence quotient is assessed on the basis of a large number of different skills. Although the general tendency is for all these skills to develop to a similar level in each individual, there can be large discrepancies, especially in people with learning disabilities. Therefore the overall category of mild, moderate or severe learning disability should be based on global assessments of ability and not on any single area of specific impairment or skill. The IQ should be determined from standardised, individually administered intelligence tests for which local cultural norms have been determined, and the test selected should be appropriate to the individual's level of functioning and additional specific handicapping conditions such as expressive language problems.

THE IMPORTANCE OF CULTURE

Cultural and religious issues are very important. They influence the value placed by society on mental health, the presentation of symptoms, illness behaviour, access to services, pathways through care, the way individuals and families manage illness, the way the community responds to illness, the degree of acceptance and support experienced by the person with mental illness, and the degree of stigma and discrimination experienced by the person with mental illness. Therefore, cultural and other contextual issues are very important to take into account in developing locally appropriate mental health policies and services.

However, there are also important similarities across different cultures. It was once thought that mental illness in general was rare in low-income countries, and that it only arose in Western cultures. A wide range of epidemiological studies over the last 40 years have demonstrated that this is not the case. Similarly, it was once thought that schizophrenia in particular was rare in low-income countries, but we now know from international epidemiological studies that the incidence of schizophrenia is similar everywhere, although there are well-replicated findings of some significant variation in the course and outcome of schizophrenia across countries and cultures which involves a higher rate of symptomatic recovery and a lower rate of social deterioration in traditional rural communities. While depression in low-income countries often presents with somatic symptoms rather than low mood (Patel et al., 1995; Abas & Broadhead, 1997), depression in Western countries also frequently presents with a high degree of somatisation (Simon et al., 1999).

Culture bound syndromes

While the above principal categories of mental disorder are found everywhere, there are a few culture-specific disorders whose status is uncertain and it is argued that they are local variations of acute anxiety and reactions to stress (WHO, 1993).

- *Amok* (Indonesia, Malaysia). An indiscriminate, seemingly unprovoked episode of homicidal or highly destructive behaviour followed by amnesia or fatigue. Many episodes culminate in suicide. May derive from traditional values placed on extreme aggression and suicidal attacks in warfare.
    Potentially related syndromes: Ahade idzi be (New Guinea), *Benzi mazurazura* (southern Africa – Shona), *Berserkagang* (Scandinavia),

Cafard (Polynesia), *Colerina* (Andes), *Hwa-byung* (Korean peninsula), *iich'aa* (indigenous peoples of south-western USA).

- *Dhat* (India, China). Anxiety and somatic complaints such as fatigue and muscle pain, related to a fear of semen loss.
- *Koro* (South East Asia, China, India). Acute panic or anxiety about fear of genital retraction.
- *Latah* (Indonesia, Malaysia). Dissociative state following fright or trauma.
- *Nerfiza, nerves, nevra, nervios* (Egypt, northern Europe, Greece, Mexico, central and southern America). Chronic episodes of extreme sorrow or anxiety with many somatic complaints.

CHAPTER TWO

The public health burden of mental illness

Key Points

- *The global burden of neuropsychiatric disorders is estimated to be increasing from 10.5% of the world's total Disability Adjusted Life Years to 15% in the year 2020.*
- *Neuropsychiatric disorders account for five out of the ten leading causes of disability.*
- *Mentally ill people face large economic and social disadvantage.*
- *A needs assessment is required in each country to underpin the development of mental health policy.*

DISABILITY ADJUSTED LIFE YEARS

Dramatic changes in the overall health needs of the world's populations are occurring. It has been generally assumed that in the developing regions, where four-fifths of the world's people live, the leading causes of disease burden are communicable diseases. In fact non-communicable diseases such as depression and heart disease are replacing the traditional enemies such as infectious diseases and malnutrition as the leading causes of disability and premature death.

Looking first at disability, psychiatric disorders account for five of the ten leading causes of disability as measured by years of life lived with a disability (Murray & Lopez, 1996). They are unipolar depression, alcohol abuse, bipolar affective disorder, schizophrenia and obsessive–compulsive disorder. Unipolar depression accounts for nearly 11% of the years lived with a disability. Alcohol use was the fourth largest cause of disability in men. Moreover, psychiatric and neurological disorders account for 28% of years of life lived with disability (Murray & Lopez, 1996). They are important contributors to years of life lived with disability in all world regions except sub-Saharan Africa (Murray & Lopez, 1996).

Secondly, looking at mortality, neuropsychiatric disorders are responsible for over 1% of all deaths. Officially recorded suicide is the tenth leading cause of death and is comparable to deaths from road traffic accidents, but many suicides are not officially registered as such, so the actual suicide rate is substantially higher than the official rate in all countries. Changes in population demography, with an increase in elderly individuals, will increase the burden due to dementia in both developed and developing countries (Shah et al., 2000; Jenkins, 1997).

Thirdly, efforts have been made to combine morbidity, disability and mortality into a single metric of the Disability Adjusted Life Year (DALY) to measure the Global Burden of Disease. Thus the Global Burden of Disease has been assessed by combining the loss of healthy life from premature death with the loss of healthy life from disability to form the quantitative Disability Adjusted Life Years (Murray, 1994; Murray & Lopez, 1996, Murray et al., 1994). The first such estimate reported in *Investing in Health* (World Bank, 1993) calculated that the global burden of neuropsychiatric disorders was 8.1% (as measured by Disability Adjusted Life Years). This has since been revised upwards to 10.5% for the world (Murray & Lopez, 1996), but across the world this figure is variable as illustrated in Table 2.1. The overall DALYs burden for developing countries due to neuropsychiatric disorders is 9% (Murray & Lopez, 1996). Unipolar depression accounts for 3.4% of DALYs in the developing world. The overall DALYs burden is projected to increase to 15% by the year 2020 for neuropsychiatric disorders – an increase that is proportionately larger than that for cardiovascular diseases (Murray & Lopez, 1996).

TABLE 2.1
The burden of neuropsychiatric disorders in each region of the world

Region	Percentage [DALYs]
Sub-Saharan Africa	4%
India	7%
China	14.2%
Latin America and Caribbean	15.9%
Middle East	8.7%
Other Asia and Islands	10.8%
Former socialist economies of Europe	17.2%
Established market economies	25.1%
Developing countries as a whole	9%
The world as a whole	10.5%

Source: Murray & Lopez (1996).

The estimates of Disability Adjusted Life Years shown in the table have made a major contribution to the very complex arguments about the relative priority of different illnesses and their morbidity and mortality by allowing morbidity, disability and mortality to be combined into a single measure. If countries are to enter the global economy, they need a strong healthy and productive workforce, and the DALY metric enables examination of how resources might be targeted in a cost-effective way.

Deficiencies of DALYs

Despite the importance of DALYs in highlighting the burden of psychiatric disorders, there are a number of important deficiencies with respect to their derivation and enumeration:

- The results, particularly in developing regions, are based on inadequate epidemiological data (particularly rates of prevalence, detection and treatment), and there is an urgent need to gather more detailed data in developing countries.
- The estimates did not include all psychiatric conditions and took no account of co-morbidity.
- The disability severity weights were specified and derived by health care experts alone, which casts doubt on the validity of both the conceptualisation of disability used and the valuation base adopted.
- They do not include estimates of family burden and under social costs.
- There is currently little indication on a practical level of how DALYs are to be linked to cost-effectiveness for improved health care decision-making and priority-setting.

If it is assumed that the DALY is to remain an influential metric in international health care policy, there are strong grounds for responding to these limitations by providing improved estimates of the disability associated with mental disorders and offering a framework for the use of DALYs in improved resource allocation.

Other measurements

Epidemiological studies conducted in Western countries have shown that up to one-fifth or one-quarter of the general population suffer from some sort of mental disorder at a given time (Weissman et al., 1978; Mavreas et al., 1986, Vazquez-Barquero et al., 1981, 1991; Jenkins et al., 1998; Bijl, 1997). Parry (1996), reviewing epidemiological studies in Africa, found similar or higher levels of morbidity, while Patel (2000), in a recent review of epidemiological studies in South East Asia, has found highly variable rates, with one study reporting a rate of 66% among women living in a poor rural area of Pakistan (Mumford et al., 1997).

Apart from their contribution to specific mental disorders, psychological factors also contribute to specific risky behaviours, which add significantly to the overall disease burden. These risky behaviours include excessive alcohol consumption, unsafe sex and tobacco use. Unsafe sex and alcohol each contribute approximately 3.5% of the total disease burden, and tobacco use contributes a further 3%. They are comparable to the burdens produced by tuberculosis and measles. In addressing poor mental health, we can also therefore address a range of physical health risks and diseases (see the section on mental health promotion in Chapter 1).

It is vital therefore that the range, frequency, severity and duration of both mental disorders and specific risky behaviours, their accompanying social disability, their mortality and their relationship with socio-demographic disorders are taken into account in health policy and planning at national level.

SOCIAL AND ECONOMIC CONSEQUENCES OF MENTAL DISORDER

Psychiatric disorders impose a significant burden in developed and developing countries. The link between poverty and mental illness is incontrovertible. The national psychiatric morbidity surveys of 1993/94 in Great Britain showed that people with any form of mental disorder had an average income of only 46.5% of the average income for the general population. In countries where there are no social security payments, as is the case in many developing countries, this situation is greatly aggravated. In addition to this effect of poverty on the individual, there is the loss of production to the economy through people with mental illness being unable to work, either in the short, medium or long term. There is also reduced productivity through people being ill while at work.

There is the socio-economic impact of the family burden, including the cost of supporting the dependents of people with mental illness. There are also long-term consequences of unemployment, crime and violence in young people whose childhood problems (e.g. depression, conduct disorder, dyslexia, other special educational needs) were not properly addressed in childhood.

Poor mental health is a risk factor for many physical health problems and emotional distress makes people more vulnerable to physical illness. Depression increases the risk of heart disease four-fold, even when other risk factors like smoking are involved (Hippisley-Cox et al., 1998). Lack of control at work is also associated with increased risk of cardiovascular disease (Bosma et al., 1997), and sustained stress or trauma increases susceptibility to viral infection and physical illness by damaging the immune system (Marmot et al., 1991; Stewart-Brown, 1998).

NEEDS ASSESSMENT

In implementing health services in developing countries, the first priority (basic hygiene and nutrition) is usually given to diseases with a high mortality rate (e.g. TB, malaria, smallpox). The next priority is generally assigned to the prevention of debilitating diseases, and the third priority (attention to the quality of life) is approached after the life expectancy has increased. Psychiatric treatment is usually tackled as part of this third category, which is surprising and illogical given the high mortality rate from suicide and associated physical illness (Harris & Barraclough, 1998) and the disability directly attributable to major mental disorders (Carstairs, 1973; Giel & Harding, 1976).

Mental health policy should be rooted in and supported by accurate information about the health and social care needs of the country, either by using national surveys of psychiatric morbidity or by extrapolation from a combination of local surveys, together with national surveys from other countries. This will be necessary to obtain accurate estimates of the range, frequency, severity, chronicity and accompanying disability and mortality and their relationship to socio-demographic variables including geographic variables (Jenkins, 2001b). The importance of covering social care and health care needs together in an integrated way cannot be overemphasised.

National surveys need to collect information on variations in local need to help to determine those areas that need more resources per capita. They can provide some comparative information which can be helpful to local areas, and they can provide help for local needs assessment (Jenkins et al., 1997a, 1997b; Meltzer et al., 1995a–c, 1995a–d; Wing, 1992). Mental health policy will also need to take into account information about the existing accessibility, quality, quantity, costs and outcomes of services (Jenkins & Knapp, 1996; Glover & Gould, 1996; Griffiths et al., 1992; Johnson et al., 1996). Furthermore, it will need to take account of the existing resource infrastructure of the country in terms of the available capital, revenue, trained personnel and untrained staff in the context of managing any kind of transition to a new style service. Other inputs, such as public beliefs and opinions, publicity about specific incidents and the political inclinations of governing parties, are crucial.

Local needs assessment

When local health planners are assessing the health needs of their local population, they will need to consider:

- *The epidemiological evidence* – both national and local – on prevalence of the different disorders, their severity and chronicity. The consequences of mental disorders will also become more salient in determining need for services and specific actions, particularly disability, and the degree of risk to self and others.

- *The policy context* – again, at both national and local levels.
- *The current levels of in-patient and residential provision* – and the existing pressures on them. In particular, they need to examine:
  - *the provision of health and social care* – the extent to which such care is being provided to people with mental illness;
  - *inter-agency working* – the extent to which there are problems with the interfaces between the different agencies providing health and social care, the criminal justice system, etc.
- *Local suicide rates.* It will be important to examine these (both those officially identified by the coroner and the 'undetermined' deaths that are likely to be suicides).
- *The physical health needs of people with mental illness.* People with severe mental illness have high standardised mortality ratios from physical illness such as cardiovascular disease, malignancy and respiratory disease (Harris and Barraclough, 1998). Therefore it is important to assess and meet their physical health needs – particularly in low-income countries where infectious diseases are rife, and the combination of poor diet, mental illness, and long-term pheno-thiazines can make patients particularly vulnerable. Hypothermia is also a problem in poor countries with a cold climate (e.g. in Eastern Europe).
- *Other variables contributing to high rates of morbidity in local areas.* These include social deprivation; urbanicity; and the combination of deprived inner city areas, marital breakdown, family breakdown, single-person households, single-parent families, unemployment and levels of substance abuse. The presence of major rail termini within a service catchment area can aggravate the effects of the geographical drift of people with severe mental illness from more rural areas to inner city areas.
- *Particular markers of high mental health needs.* These include high proportions of homeless people, alienated minority communities of different ethnic origin from the majority population, refugees, children 'at risk', children 'in care', young males aged 15–25, and people who are single, divorced or widowed. Some of these variables may be influenced by public policy and general economic developments while others may be influenced by health and social interventions.
- *Potential pressures on specialist services.* There are likely to be pre-existing heavy pressures in the following areas: secure provision for mentally disordered offenders, acute beds, 24-hour nursed care for new long-stay patients, supported housing, occupational rehabilitation,

mother and baby units, eating disorder services and drug and alcohol services.

- *The need for primary health care.* This is necessary in order to:
  - tackle the less severe disorders;
  - deliver physical health promotion and physical health care to people with mental illness;
  - contribute as locally agreed in a shared care programme for people with severe mental illness; and
  - deliver primary prevention to high-risk groups such as the socially isolated, bereaved, physically disabled, unemployed and elderly.

Local planners should ask themselves whether there is equity in their existing service provision, with people from different geographic areas, cultures, social class and the homeless all having their needs met equitably. They need to know the costs that are associated with the current provision, the obstacles that currently exist to planning co-ordinated and comprehensive services, and how the services might be improved.

CHAPTER THREE

Developing the overall strategy

Key Points

- *Each country will require its own mental health strategy.*
- *Key agencies must be identified and engaged.*
- *A common strategic framework for mental health, applicable in all countries, is set out.*
- *Implementation is even more challenging than strategy formulation and key implementation issues are also set out.*
- *Joined-up policy-making is required across government.*

Mental health policy is increasingly a focus of long overdue attention in many countries. This is partly due to the impetus within the mental health field itself from service users, their families and mental health professionals; and partly because of the illogicality of conducting general health sector reforms without paying due attention to a significant portion of the health services.

If the public health burden of mental illness is to be tackled effectively, it is necessary for governments to adopt a strategic approach that encompasses much more than just curative services for acutely ill people. Most countries focus their policy efforts on the specialist services, but this ignores the fact that the overall mental health care system is extremely complex, comprising many different agencies which inevitably come into contact with people with mental illness, and the interfaces and patient-flows through the system will inevitably have consequences for the rest of the system. For example, it is very difficult to resettle people with severe mental illness in the community if the stigma surrounding people with mental illness is not tackled through public education in schools and communities. Similarly, it is impossible for relatively scarce specialists to focus on people with severe mental illness if they are constantly deluged by large volumes of referrals of mildly or moderately ill people.

Each country has special needs, problems, resource constraints and challenges. Nevertheless, however constrained a country may be for resources, there are some consistent and interdependent areas that each country's national strategy needs to address if it is to make most effective use of available resources to improve the mental health of its people.

DETERMINING THE NEXT STEPS IN A MENTAL HEALTH STRATEGY

No organisation or government starts strategy development with a blank sheet of paper. Each will start from its own information base, from the context of its overall health and social policy, and within its own social history and its own mix of stakeholders and stakeholder views. This is why strategy development is best done nationally, by the responsible agencies – solutions cannot be imported on the back of a lorry. However, there are certain principles in mental health strategy development, which may be of general help and applicability.

General management models of strategy development are centrally relevant to mental health. This section relies heavily on Bryson's analysis (Bryson, 1995), as this is specifically addressed to a public policy environment, but other analyses are helpful. Most readers will be familiar with the public policy cycle, which goes through formulation, implementation and evaluation, which in turn feeds back into reformulation. Bryson extends this model into ten key steps, all of which are relevant to mental health. They are set out in Box 3.1.

BOX 3.1
Bryson's ten steps to strategic planning (adapted)

1. Initiate and agree the strategic planning process.
2. Identify relevant organisational roles and mandates.
3. Identify the mission and the values.
4. Carry out SWOT analysis (Strengths, Weaknesses, Opportunities, Threats) and a needs analysis or assemble existing data.
5. Identify the key strategic issues.
6. Formulate the strategy.
7. Adopt strategic plan.
8. Establish the vision.
9. Implement the plan.
10. Reassess the strategy.

Steps 1 and 2: What is the process and who are the stakeholders?

Steps 1 and 2 are probably best undertaken in tandem. The individual or organisation which is taking the lead needs to assemble a list of the interested parties and agencies and agree with the key players what the planning process is going to be, how long it will take and how they will be consulted. It is important to identify all the key agencies with an interest – otherwise agencies that could help (or hinder) the plan could be missed. Box 3.2 gives a list of the categories into which the key agencies might fall.

It is worth carrying out a brief analysis of the role and potential role of each agency in relation to mental health. This will vary from country to country. There may, for example, be certain industries with very high rates

BOX 3.2
Types of agency with an interest in mental health

1. *The general public and people with mental illness and their carers.*

2. *Public bodies*
   – The Health Ministry
   – Other government ministries such as Social Welfare, Employment, Education, Home Affairs/Criminal Justice, Environment/Housing, Information and Tourism
   – Public health care agencies
   – Health promotion/health education agencies
   – Social services
   – Social welfare/benefits agencies
   – Employment rehabilitation services
   – Housing agencies
   – The police, prisons and criminal justice agencies
   – Schools and higher education institutions.

3. *Private business*
   – Insurance companies
   – Private health care companies
   – The pharmaceutical industry
   – Business generally, especially employers' organisations.

4. *Churches/organised religion*
   – National and local religious leaders
   – Religious social and health care institutions.

5. *The voluntary sector* (non-governmental organisations)
   – Mental health and health care organisations
   – Organisations concerned with poverty, youth, old age
   – Human rights and other relevant issues.

6. *The media.*

7. *Professional bodies.*

of mental illness, or a certain product which is favoured for self-harm or suicide, in which case the industry or manufacturer concerned needs to be engaged with the strategy.

It will be uncertain that all the major stakeholders will agree that a strategy is necessary or desirable, and a communications exercise may be necessary to engage them. Different stakeholders may require different arguments. Industry and the taxpayer may need to be confronted with the economic burdens, and professionals and government may need information on proven effectiveness and epidemiology. Historically, human rights and ethical arguments have also been of great importance in moving mental health services forward. Good-quality public affairs and public relations advice on how to prepare the ground for a mental health strategy is worth having from an early stage.

The views of service users and carers will be particularly important, given that they will be directly affected by the implementation of the strategy and will have personal experience of the problems in the current system. They will also be able to comment on those aspects of the current mental health system that are working well.

Ways of gaining mental health service user views and involving them

This will vary from country to country. Box 3.3 sets out some possible ways of gaining the views of service users, and many of these options apply equally to carers.

The consequences of not involving service users and reasons why the user voice is often ineffective (and how to address this) are discussed in Chapter 15 (Common problems).

BOX 3.3
Involving service users in the development of the strategy

- Hold national or local opinion surveys or focus groups.
- Facilitate the formation of national and local user organisations which will be autonomous and self-sustaining.
- Seek the assistance of existing NGOs in facilitating user involvement.
- Recruit service users on to national and local advisory groups, boards, etc.
- Encourage user involvement in quality assurance, including national inspection agencies and in the determination of quality standards.
- Promote advocacy schemes to support user involvement as well as the defence of individual user rights.
- Engage (and remunerate) user consultants to undertake specific tasks where their contribution is key, including training of professionals in the user perspective.
- Ensure that policy-makers meet regularly with users to take their views.

Step 3: What is the mission?

This is not easy as the different stakeholders may have very different ideas on what mental health services should do. However, no strategy will succeed unless a critical mass of stakeholders are satisfied or at least compliant. It is therefore worth carrying out a stakeholder analysis to determine (a) stakeholders' key interests and (b) what they are likely to want from a mental health strategy. Although there will undoubtedly be a need for leadership, the strategy has to take account of stakeholder views, in particular the views of the service users. The overall goals of public policy on mental health generally include some or all of the elements listed in Box 3.4.

The mission also needs to take account of the assessment of the current situation and local priorities, for example, emphasising the needs of specific groups such as women and children. Health-oriented missions are possibly less useful than broader ones which emphasise social functioning and social care as well as health care.

BOX 3.4
Possible elements for a mental health mission

1. To reduce the incidence and prevalence of mental illness.
2. To reduce mortality associated with mental illness.
3. To reduce the extent and severity of problems associated with specific mental disorders, including poor health and social functioning.
4. To develop mental health services.
5. To promote good mental health and reduce stigma.
6. To protect the human rights and dignity of mentally ill people.

Step 4: The SWOT analysis and the needs analysis

The SWOT analysis (see Box 3.4) and the needs assessment (see Chapter 2) together form the analysis of the environment in which planning is going to take place. They can be undertaken using a range of techniques, but it is important to draw together both the facts and some analysis of those facts. The overall environmental analysis can be done in a number of ways, but the SWOT technique, which is one of the most common, involves listing out the major features of the planning environment. Box 3.5 contains some headings, which could be considered in the SWOT analysis with examples.

In carrying out the SWOT analysis it is worth spending quite a bit of time on the opportunities as these are likely to be very country-specific (hence

BOX 3.5
The SWOT analysis: a mental health framework

Strengths
- Who is committed to the mission?
- Are there good signs in the epidemiology (e.g. areas of low prevalence, or areas of declining prevalence)?
- Are there protective factors (family/society)?
- What are the strengths of mental health services now?
- What are the strengths of other relevant services including primary care?
- Are there generic mechanisms within society, which are relevant, e.g. education, religion, etc.?
- What is the attitude of the media?
- What useful resources are there (money/staff/networks)?

Weaknesses
- Who may be opposed?
- What are the epidemiological warning signs?
- Are there vulnerability factors?
- What are the weaknesses of mental health services?
- What are the weaknesses of other relevant services, including primary care?
- Is the system able to deliver?
- What building blocks are missing?

Opportunities
- Who is ready to move?
- Are there pots of resource available?
- Is outside help available?
- Is the health care system being reformed/developed?
- Is awareness increasing?
- Are there human resources already available that could be deployed to support the strategy?
- Are there continuing education budgets to be accessed?
- Are there individuals in primary care with psychiatric training?
- Are there pre-existing health promotion programmes (e.g. alcohol and drugs) which are relevant?

Threats
- Are other priorities perceived as more important?
- Are budgets being cut?
- Is the ideological climate worsening?
- Are essential contributors under threat (e.g. primary care, medical education)?
- Are there any major political changes or national disasters?

the limited list of suggestions) and may be most helpful to strategy formulation. Many of the threats and weaknesses will be self-evident.

Step 5: The key strategic issues

Once the SWOT analysis has been carried out, the key strategic issues will become clearer. At this stage it is suggested that a more detailed analysis could be drawn up consisting of three columns: strategic area for action, expected results, and consequences of not acting. This will clarify priorities and will help to convince others of the value of the strategy. Box 3.6 suggests a more detailed common strategic framework for mental health, with expected results and consequences of inaction for each item.

Step 6: Formulating the strategy

Only at this stage does detailed strategy formulation start. The strategy, in essence, needs to consist of a statement of the key objectives and the major actions that will take place to achieve those objectives. In addition, most strategies include information about time-scale, costs, milestones and targets, evaluation and action leads, either in the strategic plan, or more commonly in an associated operational plan. But all this material is subordinate to the description of the objectives and to the actions that will be taken to achieve the desired outcomes.

The strategy must flow naturally from the preceding analysis and should be realistic given the nation's starting point and the degree to which the local population is scattered over large rural areas. For example, most if not all countries will need to develop the primary care of common mental disorders in any event. Thus, questions which will need to be considered are as follows:

- Is there currently a primary care system across the country and, if so, what cadres of professionals does it contain (doctors, nurses, medical assistants, health workers)?
- Have professionals received any mental health tuition in their basic training, and could this be reinforced by a programme of continuing education and use of good practice guidelines?
- Is there a system of specialist supervision and quality control in primary care?

The precise tasks that may be assigned to primary care will depend on these factors and on the extent to which there is specialist capacity for referral. For the care of people with severe mental illness, a capital-led strategy to build and sustain a large number of local in-patient facilities and train large numbers of expensive specialists will be beyond the means

Box 3.6
A common strategic framework for mental health

Task	Results	Consequences of inaction
1. Develop a mental health promotion strategy embracing generic settings such as schools, the workplace, urban and rural areas.	Increased understanding of mental health and mental ill health, routine action to protect mental health, early presentation of problems, reduced morbidity, reduced economic burden.	Continued stigma, lack of presentation, steady or increasing economic burden.
2. Develop mental health legislation, which protects human rights and controls the circumstances in which patients can be held in hospital or treated without consent.	Human rights are protected. Compliance with international treaties.	Rights may be violated. Negative campaigning may be encouraged. Poor public relations. Risk of national or international legal challenge.
3. Educate, support and resource primary care in its essential role of tackling the majority of people with mental health problems.	Efficiency. Sensitivity to patient and the community. Cost-effectiveness. Raised morale in primary care. Good outcomes for mild–moderate disorders (which nonetheless impose huge burdens).	Primary care swamped with untreated mental health problems and somatisation. Inefficient pattern of onward referrals. Inefficiency. Poor morale. Poor outcomes.
4. Develop effective links between primary and secondary care including social care, with well-developed criteria for referral, methods of shared care, adequate information systems and communication, etc.	Similar to 1. Secondary care functions with maximum efficiency.	Poor functioning of secondary care. Inefficiency. Patients fall through the gaps – sometimes with serious consequences.

5. Configure or reconfigure the mental health infrastructure to develop comprehensive local specialist health and social services which have good inter-agency working with other key agencies (e.g. NGOs, criminal justice system).	Good outcomes. Sensitivity to need. Patients can occupy least restrictive and most cost-effective slot in the system.	Patients may 'block' any in-patient facilities, as they have nowhere to move to. Others will get inadequate care. Poor outcomes. Poor sensitivity to need. Inefficiency.
6. Develop good practice guidelines on effective interventions in primary and secondary care, and on inter-agency working.	Efficiency. Good communications. Avoids a variety of inconsistent local practices springing up. Stops patients dropping out of the system.	Use of ineffective interventions. Poor communications. Patients being lost to service support and follow up, with consequent relapse and increased disability.
7. Develop a package of public health measures to reduce mental ill health, suicides and homicides by mentally ill people.	Reduced mortality. Increased public confidence. Efficient (public health measures are often more cost-effective than secondary care interventions).	Health care services may be overwhelmed. Loss of public confidence. Unnecessary deaths.
8. Develop a research and development strategy for mental health.	Improved efficiency and effectiveness. Better informed staff. Better services.	Decay in the quality and effectiveness of services. Services unable to keep pace with global research findings. Lack of innovation. Services frozen into outdated models.
9. Consider the mental health impact of all general policy and general health and social care policy.	Co-ordinated approach Synergy between policies gives added value with budgets.	Avoidance of perverse outcomes from policy. Avoidance of inefficiency, duplication.

of many nations. A community-based strategy for people with severe mental illness, perhaps with unqualified workers supervised by professionals, tailored to the strength of local family support systems and the degree of assumption of responsibilities for sick family members, may be possible. Alternatively, it may be best for the small number of available specialists to tackle more severe mental illness, and to support primary care to address the remainder.

There is usually little merit in completely overthrowing existing systems – an evolutionary approach is often most cost-effective and feasible. Sometimes, however, elements of the existing system may be so poor that it is easiest to start again. For example, old mental hospitals with totally inadequate premises and institutionalised staff might have to be closed. In many cases, the strategy will need to concentrate more on creating a framework for investment and development, rather than detailing exactly who the providers will be – as this will probably come later.

The time-scale will also be an important part of the strategy. Five to ten years is probably a realistic period to achieve significant change. Any shorter time-scale is likely to be unrealistic, while too long a time horizon may leave many stakeholders cold and inactive. Different elements of the strategy may require different time-scales; for example:

- Reconfigure old long-stay hospital service into a comprehensive locally based service: 20–30 years.
- Close a single hospital: 5 years.
- Establish an occupational rehabilitation project: 3 years.
- Reform professional training and establish national accreditation procedures: 5 years.
- Train psychiatrists: 10 years (5–6 years basic medical training and five years post-qualification training and experience).
- Establish basic training for unqualified workers: 3 years.
- Reform mental health legislation: 3 years.
- Establish an R&D strategy: 2 years, 5 years for first results.
- Establish a health care information system: 3 years.
- Start a national mental health promotion programme: 2 years.
- Roll out good practice protocols in primary and secondary care: 2 years.
- Restrict access to a means of suicide: 1–2 years.

Steps 7 and 8: Adopt the strategy and establish the vision

It is much easier to write a strategic plan than it is to have it adopted or implemented. Adoption involves getting approval, crucially from government, but no less crucially from the other key stakeholders. This process is likely to require strong advocacy and strong arguments. It is important to stress both the benefits of action – such as, improved national mental health, lower economic burdens and improved human rights – together with the possible negative consequences. Wherever possible, hard epidemiological and economic data should be used to support the case.

It is worth considering developing a separate communications strategy to support the principal strategy. Communication is a cross-cutting theme, which underpins all work in mental health. There is great value, for example, in placing both positive and negative media stories about the inadequacies of current policy and services and what could be achieved if change proceeded. This can often be done without conflict of interest by non-governmental organisations (NGOs). It is also essential to have some well-placed product champions to advocate the strategy at the highest levels within government and other key agencies. The ideal strategy in a business, medical and scientific sense will not succeed unless mental health is pushed up the governmental agenda, and this rarely happens by chance.

In establishing the vision it is also vitally important to communicate the strategy to all the partner agencies and, within those agencies, to individuals. Many strategies fail simply because of poor communication. Either they are not communicated at all, or the essence of the strategy is missed and people become obsessed with contentious details that are not essential to the overall vision.

Step 9: Implementation

As already stated, the strategic plan will need to be associated with an operational plan, or have operational elements embedded within it. It needs to describe who does what, by when and with what resources. The principles of implementation are well described in the management literature. Some issues that are of particular relevance to mental health are listed in Box 3.7.

Step 10: Review

It is useful to build in a formal review point for the strategy, perhaps after three or five years. At this stage there should be some data available to enable outcomes, or at least outputs, to be assessed along with stakeholder views. The key questions to ask are:

- What has worked?
- Can we do more of it?

BOX 3.7
Implementation issues for mental health strategies

1. *Communications*
   - Public relations
   - Public affairs
   - Cascading information within organisations
   - Organising feedback
   - Alliance building – targeting key partners
   - Maintaining the profile of the strategy with opinion formers
   - Keeping product champions on board
   - Publicising success
   - Managing failures.

2. *Resources*
   - Accessing key budgets
   - Securing capital, including private sector venture capital
   - Ensuring revenue flows
   - Maximising the use of generic budgets
   - Sponsorship and aid.

3. *Staff*
   - Planning the development of the human resource
   - Re-skilling for changing service configurations
   - Basic and continuing education for mental health staff
   - Skilling generic staff (e.g. primary care, teachers) on mental health
   - Communicating with staff
   - Engaging professional bodies and educational institutions
   - Using unskilled staff efficiently.

4. *Embedding the strategy*
   - Engaging generic organisations, managers, politicians
   - Disseminating good practice
   - Implementing an R&D strategy, including evaluation
   - Learning from mistakes and successes and fine tuning the strategy
   - Quality assurance, accreditation and inspection.

- What has not worked?
- Can we fine tune?
- Can we invest the resource elsewhere?
- What elements are we uncertain about?
- How do we improve evaluation so that we will know whether the various elements of the strategy are working?

No strategy will ever be definitive over time because the environment and the epidemiology will evolve – all strategies must be dynamic.

Linking the strategy across policies and government departments

As already stated, the mental health strategy needs to be linked in with generic health policy and across government policies generally. It is particularly important that any general public health strategy addresses mental as well as physical health so that:

- mortality indicators include suicides (with attention to enhancing the accuracy of recording of suicides);
- morbidity indicators include, or plan to include, relevant measures of morbidity due to mental illness;
- public health interventions in areas such as housing and social welfare are assessed for their impact on mental health;
- any health impact assessments or statements or similar measures explicitly include mental health.

GENERAL GOVERNMENT POLICIES

In order to achieve these goals, the government sectors that are able to influence mental health – which include health social welfare, employment, trade and industry, education (both schools and higher education institutions), home affairs, police, prisons and criminal justice agencies, environment and housing, and finance (see Box 3.8) – must be engaged. The settings for action include workplaces, schools, prisons, cities, rural areas, health services and social services. Other agencies with an interest in mental health include:

- private business – insurance companies, private health care companies
- the pharmaceutical industry
- business generally, especially employers' organisations
- places of worship and organised religion, including national and local religious leaders, religious social and health care institutions (which in some countries form the backbone of the health care provision)
- organisations concerned with poverty, youth, old age, human rights, and other relevant issues
- the voluntary sector, non-governmental organisations
- user and carer groups.

Governments need to ensure (a) that all relevant agencies are aware of the importance of mental health for the population, (b) that they are aware of the influence that their activities can have on mental health, and (c) that appropriate co ordination between relevant agencies takes place. This co-ordination is often in place for action on alcohol and drugs, and for AIDS programmes, but is as yet rarely in place for mental health programmes, despite mental illness forming the greater burden across the population.

The following specific areas should be considered by certain government departments:

- *The Ministry of Employment, Trade and Industry* needs to consider access to employment, including sheltered employment, employment rehabilitation, workplace mental health policies, and occupational health of the workforce in order to support a successful economy and play its role in the prevention of discrimination.

- *The Ministry of Education* needs to include education on mental health as part of the health and social skills elements of school curricula, and to develop the higher education appropriate for the country's needs, including generic courses, vocational qualifications, distance learning, and occupational standards relevant to mental health.

- *The Ministry of Home Affairs* needs to ensure both public security and the welfare of mentally ill people in contact with the police and the prisons, usually by appropriate diversion from the criminal justice system into the health system. There may need to be collaboration on the provision of secure treatment facilities for the very small number of highly dangerous mentally disordered offenders. The Ministry of Home Affairs will also need to address the relative availability of alcohol and other addictive substances, and to consider appropriate measures such as taxation to keep the price of alcohol artificially inflated, and controls to limit the supply of illicit substances which contribute to mental illness and frequently aggravate psychotic mental illness and psychotic episodes.

- *The Ministry of the Environment and Housing* will need to consider the impact of its planning decisions on the mental as well as the physical health of the population, and to consider the needs for sheltered housing for people with severe mental illness if they cannot live with their families. An adequate supply of housing is an important contributor to mental health, and there is plenty of evidence of the detrimental effect of being homeless or housed in crowded temporary accommodation. Homelessness is particularly problematic in cold countries and there can be a strong correlation between homelessness and mental health problems.

- *The Ministry for Women* will need to consider access to education, training and health care for women, and the influence of other government policies on these issues. It will need to liaise with other government departments, particularly the Ministry for Home Affairs, on government policies influencing family cohesiveness, for example, mechanisms such as taxation and welfare benefits in place to support families, reduce family breakdown, and reduce the burden on women as they struggle to raise their children. In some countries, mental illness is a sufficient reason for divorce, and such premature divorces will often leave a parent without financial support, to the detriment of the mother and child. It is therefore important to make available marital support and therapy. This is an activity that can often be usefully delivered by an NGO.

- *The Ministry of Health* will need to consider not just policy for specialist services but, even more importantly, policy for primary care where most people with mental disorder are cared for and where many opportunities for prevention and early detection exist. It will need to pay attention to professional education and human resources, to methods of financing training and service delivery, to public health strategy, to client group policies and to the occupational health of the health care workforce if it is to safeguard its investment in training. The social care agenda for mental health is also vitally important and needs to be tied in to the strategy whether social care policy is placed with the Ministry of Health or elsewhere.

- *The Ministry of Social Welfare* will need to consider mental health in its legislation on disability, anti-discrimination and any welfare benefits. It needs to consider the mental as well as the physical health and development of children in its care. Records show that a large proportion of people in prison have previously been in children's homes and orphanages.

- *The Ministry of Finance* will need to ensure adequate funding for the above programmes.

To summarise, governments need to ensure that all relevant agencies are aware of the importance of mental health for their population, that they are aware of the influence their policies and activities can have on the mental health of the population, and that appropriate co-ordination between relevant agencies takes place.

It is therefore essential that every country creates a strategic mental health policy which is well integrated with its general public policies and with its overall health policy at ministerial, ministry, regional and local levels, and which covers the three broad tasks:

- community action to promote mental health;
- primary care of mental disorders for prevention and prompt and efficient treatment of common mental disorders; and
- specialist services (as local as is affordable) to support those clients in greatest need and to support and sustain expertise in primary care.

BOX 3.8
Policy links for the mental health strategy

1. *Health Department*
   - Primary care policy
   - Human resources, professional training, continuing education
   - Finance
   - Commissioning and providing models
   - Public health strategy
   - Client group (e.g. children, older people) policies
   - Occupational health of the health care workforce
   - Social care.

2. *Social Welfare*
   - Access to social welfare benefits for mentally ill people.

3. *Employment*
   - Access to employment, including sheltered employment
   - Employment rehabilitation
   - Workplace mental health policies
   - Occupational health.

4. *Education*
   - Including education on mental health as part of health and social skills elements of school curricula
   - Developing higher education including generic courses, vocational qualifications, distance learning, and occupational standards relevant to mental health
   - Training and continuing education for teachers to be able to recognise and address the special needs of children with dyslexia, emotional and conduct disorders.

5. *Home Affairs and Criminal Justice*
   - Diversion of mentally ill offenders out of the criminal justice system
   - Public security and the welfare of mentally ill people in contact with the police and criminal justice system.

6. *Environment/Housing*
   - Ensuring an adequate supply of ordinary and special needs/sheltered housing for mentally ill people.

7. *Trade and Industry*
   - Maintaining communications with insurance companies and others
   - Preventing discrimination (relevant generally).

Mental health policy needs to encompass:

- primary and secondary health and social care, the links between them, and methods of ensuring good practice;
- liaison between the health services and the social welfare services, the criminal justice system including the police and the prisons, the education system, workplaces and the general community;

- the interface between the public and the private sectors and the non-governmental sector;
- attention to some generic issues essential for the success of any health policy, such as the information strategy, the research and development strategy and the human resources strategy;
- some specific vital issues such as the precise funding streams for mental health and the organisational structure for policy implementation;
- consideration of the generic role of legislation in supporting the implementation of the mental health strategy, as well as the specific mental health legislation, to set the overall philosophy of approach to the care of people with mental disorders together with precise provision for assessment and treatment without consent under certain defined conditions in the interests of the public.

These elements are listed in Box 3.9.

BOX 3.9
The strategic framework

National components
- National strategy to promote mental health, reduce morbidity and reduce mortality
- Policy links with other government departments
- Legislation to support the national mental health policy
- Establishment of the funding streams
- Organogram for implementation and accountability.

Support infrastructure
- Mental health information strategy
- Research and development strategy
- Human resource strategy.

Service components
- Mental health promotion in schools, workplaces and the community
- Primary care
- Secondary care
- Social care
- Effective links between primary care and secondary care
- Good practice guidelines in primary health care units and out-patient clinics
- Liaison with the police
- Liaison with the prisons
- Liaison, collaboration and shared care with traditional healers
- Liaison and collaboration with NGOs.

CHAPTER FOUR

Legislation and the mental health strategy

Key Points

- *Mental health legislation has a key role in protecting human rights and in supporting the overall mental health strategy.*
- *Basic principles from international treaties and declarations are presented.*
- *Five core principles underpinning mental health legislation are identified.*
- *Seven key issues to be addressed in such legislation are described.*

THE ROLE OF LEGISLATION IN DEVELOPING A MENTAL HEALTH STRATEGY

In Chapter 3 legislation was identified as one of the 'national components of the strategic framework'. Legislation must be part of, and support, the mental health strategy. In addition to defining roles and responsibilities of agencies involved in the development and implementation of the strategy, legislation will be central to the protection of the human rights of individuals with mental illness. Thus legislation will have two distinct but interlinked roles:

- *Supporting the strategy*
  Many aspects of the mental health strategy will need to be underpinned by legislation. For example, if part of the strategy is 'To develop a comprehensive local specialist health and social services' (see Box 3.6) the agencies responsible for these services will need to establish a co-ordinated approach to care. Thus, existing legislation should be examined to ensure that any legal barriers to agencies working together are removed, or at least reduced.

41

- *Protecting human rights*
  If individuals with mental illness are to be treated and/or detained
  against their wishes, legislation must ensure that these powers may only
  be exercised in strictly defined circumstances and that adequate safeguards are included in order to prevent arbitrary interference with
  individuals' rights and freedoms.

Supporting the strategy

Box 3.2 in Chapter 3 identified the range of agencies which are likely to
have an interest in mental health. Equally, the legislative framework in
which these agencies operate is likely to have an impact on the mental
health strategy. Accordingly, existing legislation must be examined in the
light of the mental health strategy to ensure that any tensions between
the strategy and the powers and duties of the agencies can be identified
and resolved. For example:

1. If the strategy envisages that people who require treatment for their
    mental illness are diverted from the criminal justice system to appro-
    priate health care settings, the judiciary must have the power to make
    such orders. If current legislation only allows for custodial sentences
    to be made, the legislation would need to be amended to provide for
    the circumstances in which individuals may be sent to hospitals. In
    addition, legislation would aid the strategy by specifying the roles of
    the Ministry of Home Affairs and the Ministry of Health and requiring
    them to co-operate with each other in this area.
2. If attempting suicide is a criminal offence, this will conflict with any
    strategy to de-stigmatise mental illness and is likely to deter people
    who feel suicidal from seeking help. Accordingly, consideration
    should be given to repealing such a law.
3. In some countries, where the development of community-based
    services is at a very early stage, legislation may be required to create
    social care agencies. Such agencies should have the responsibility for
    arranging social services and co-ordinating with health care services,
    and other relevant agencies, at both individual and organisational
    levels.

The areas of legislation which would be relevant to the mental health
strategy include:

- housing – particularly the provision of housing to vulnerable members
  of society
- social services – particularly the responsibilities for the planning and
  provision of community-based services and how such responsibilities
  are shared with health agencies

- employment
- education
- anti-discrimination
- criminal justice.

PROTECTING HUMAN RIGHTS

One of the key elements of a mental health strategy should be to:

Develop mental health legislation which protects human rights and controls the circumstances in which patients can be held in hospital or treated without consent.

The legal framework for compulsory detention and treatment should reflect the various international human rights treaties. The three treaties, which together form the *International Bill of Human Rights*, are as follows:

- Universal Declaration of Human Rights 1948 ('the Universal Declaration'). Although this document is not legally binding on States, many of the provisions are generally considered to be part of international law because they are so widely accepted and used as a yardstick for measuring the conduct of States (United Nations, 1998: 218).
- International Covenant on Economic, Social and Cultural Rights 1976. This is legally binding on the States who have ratified it, requiring a State to take steps, to the maximum of its available resources, to achieve 'progressively the full realisation' of the rights set out in the Covenant. It includes the right to the enjoyment of the highest attainable standard of mental and physical health.
- International Covenant of Civil and Political Rights 1976. This is legally binding on the States who have ratified it, requiring them 'to respect and to ensure to all individuals' within their territory and subject to their jurisdiction the rights set out in the Covenant'. It includes the right to liberty and freedom from inhuman or degrading treatment.

Other United Nation treaties to which States may be party include the International Convention on the Elimination of Racial Discrimination (1966), the Convention Against Torture and Other Inhuman or Degrading Treatment or Punishment (1984) and the Convention on the Rights of the Child (1989). States will need to take account of their obligations under these Conventions when developing mental health legislation. For example, when considering the procedures involved in the compulsory admission of children and young people to hospital for treatment for mental illness, those States who have ratified the Convention on the Rights of the Child would need to consider the following article:

'Every child deprived of liberty shall be treated with humanity and respect for the inherent dignity of the human person, and in a manner which takes into account the needs of persons of his or her age. In particular, every child deprived of liberty shall be separated from adults unless it is considered in the child's best interest not to do so and shall have the right to maintain contact with his or her family through correspondence and visits, save in exceptional circumstances.' (Article 37c)

States will also need to consider their obligations under any regional human rights treaties to which they are party, such as the European Convention of Human Rights or the African Charter on Human and People's Rights. In addition legislation must comply with the State's own written constitution, if any.

The boxes below give examples of articles included in international and regional treaties which will be of direct relevance to legislation which provides for the involuntary admission to hospital and/or compulsory treatment of individuals.

The Right to Liberty

- *Universal Declaration of Human Rights*

  'Everyone has the right to life, liberty and security of person.' (Article 3)

  'No one shall be subjected to arbitrary arrest, detention or exile.' (Article 9)

- *International Covenant on Civil and Political Rights*

  'Everyone has the right to liberty and security of person. No one shall be subjected to arbitrary arrest or detention. No one shall be deprived of his liberty except on such grounds and in accordance with such procedure as are established by law.' (Article 9(1))

  'Anyone who is deprived of his liberty by arrest or detention shall be entitled to take proceedings before a court, in order that that court may decide without delay on the lawfulness of his detention and order his release if the detention is not lawful.' (Article 9(4))

- *European Convention on Human Rights*

  'Everyone has the right to liberty and security of person. No one shall be deprived of his liberty save in the following cases and in accordance with a procedure prescribed by law:

    'e. the lawful detention of persons for the prevention of the spreading of infectious diseases, of persons of unsound mind, alcoholics or drug addicts or vagrants [case-law has set out the conditions which must be met in order for the detention of person of 'unsound mind' to be lawful – see below].' (Article 5(1))

  'Everyone who is deprived of his liberty by arrest or detention shall be entitled to take proceedings by which the lawfulness of his detention shall be decided speedily by a court and his release ordered if the detention is not lawful.' (Article 5(4))

  Thus in order to protect this right, legislation must ensure that an individual's liberty may only be restricted in clearly defined circumstances.

Freedom from torture and inhuman treatment

- *Universal Declaration of Human Rights*

  'No one shall be subjected to torture or to cruel, inhuman or degrading treatment or punishment.' (Article 5)

- *International Covenant on Civil and Political Rights*

  'No one shall be subjected to torture or to cruel, inhuman or degrading treatment or punishment. In particular, no one shall be subjected without his free consent to medical or scientific experimentation.' (Article 7)

- *European Convention on Human Rights*

  'No one shall be subjected to torture or to inhuman or degrading treatment or punishment.' (Article 3)

  This right will be relevant to the conditions in which a person is detained and the care that he or she receives. While mental health legislation will not necessarily be directly concerned with the standard of the hospital environment, policies on seclusion and attitude of staff, these will need to be regularly monitored to ensure that individuals are not subjected to cruel, inhuman or degrading treatment. This will be particularly important for people who are compulsorily detained in mental health facilities or those who, although theoretically free to leave, are in practice unable to do so due to their incapacity.

The Right to Privacy

- *Universal Declaration of Human Rights*

  'No one shall be subjected to arbitrary interference with his privacy, family, home or correspondence, nor to attacks upon his honour and reputation. Everyone has the right to the protection of the law against such interference or attacks.' (Article 12)

- *International Covenant on Civil and Political Rights*

  'No one shall be subjected to arbitrary or unlawful interference with his privacy, family home or correspondence, nor to unlawful attacks on his honour and reputation.' (Article 17(1))

- *European Convention on Human Rights*

  '(1) Everyone has the right to respect for his private and family life, his home and his correspondence.
  (2) There shall be no interference by a public authority with the exercise of this right except such as is in accordance with the law and is necessary in a democratic society in the interests of national security, public safety or the economic well-being of the country, for the prevention of disorder or crime, for the protection of health or morals, or for the protection of the rights and freedoms of others.' (Article 8)

  The fact that a person is detained should not unnecessarily restrict his or her rights to communicate with family and friends. In order to guard against arbitrary interference with a person's right to privacy, legislation should describe the circumstances in which treatment may be given without consent. Legislation should also provide for the regular monitoring of policies on visiting, withholding mail and personal searches in addition to the exercise of compulsory treatment provisions in order to ensure that there is no undue interference with the privacy and family life of individuals.

The Right to Non-discrimination

- *Universal Declaration of Human Rights*

  'Everyone is entitled to all the rights and freedoms set forth in this Declaration without distinction of any kind, such as race, colour, sex, language, religion, political or other opinion, national or social origin, property, birth or other status.' (Article 2)

- *International Covenant on Civil and Political Rights*

  'All persons are equal before the law and are entitled without any discrimination to the equal protection of the law. In this respect the law shall prohibit any discrimination and guarantee to all persons equal and effective protection against discrimination on any ground such as race, colour, sex, language, religion, political or other opinion, national or social origin, property, birth or other status.' (Article 26)

- *European Convention on Human Rights*

  'The enjoyment of rights and freedoms set forth in this Convention shall be secured without discrimination on any ground such as sex, race, colour, language, religion, political or other opinion, national or social origin, association with a national minority, property, birth or other status.'(Article 14)

  Individuals who have a diagnosis of 'mental illness' or other condition would fall within the catch-all category 'other status'. Thus legislation must not allow the restriction of rights or freedoms simply on the basis that a person has a mental illness. In practice, however, discrimination against people with mental illness still occurs in many countries.

The United Nations has also adopted other standards relating to the protection of human rights which will be relevant to people with mental illness. These include:

- Principles for the Protection of Persons with Mental Illnesses and the Improvement of Health Care – General Assembly Resolution 46/119 of 17 December 1991 ('the UN Principles').
- Principles of Medical Ethics relevant to the Role of Health Personnel, particularly Physicians, in the Protection of Prisoners and Detainees against Torture and Other Cruel, Inhuman or Degrading Treatment or Punishment – General Assembly Resolution 37/194 of 18 December 1982.
- Body of Principles for the Protection of All Persons under Any Form of Detention or Imprisonment – General Assembly Resolution 43/173 of 9 December 1988.
- Declaration on the Rights of Mentally Retarded Persons – Proclaimed by General Resolution 2856(XXVI) of 20 December 1971.

These instruments are not treaties and are therefore not directly binding on States. However they are considered to have a significant impact given that 'they are usually carefully drafted by States and adopted by consensus' (United Nations, 1998: 223) and as such can be viewed as a guide to States on how they should interpret their obligations under the international treaties (Rosenthal & Rubenstein, 1993).

Examples of the Principles for the Protection of Persons with Mental Illnesses and the Improvement of Health Care are set out below.

Principle 1: Fundamental Freedoms and Basic Rights

1. All persons have the right to the best available mental health care, which shall be part of the health and social care system.
2. All persons with a mental illness who are to be treated as such persons, shall be treated with humanity and respect for the inherent dignity of the human person.
3. All persons with a mental illness, or who are being treated as such persons, have the right to protection from economic, sexual and other forms of exploitation, physical or other abuse and degrading treatment.

Principle 4: Determination of Mental Illness

1. The determination that a person has a mental illness shall be made in accordance with internationally accepted medical standards.

Principle 7: Role of Community and Culture

1. Every patient shall have the right to be treated and cared for, as far as possible, in the community in which he or she lives.
2. Where treatment takes place in a mental health facility, a patient shall have the right, wherever possible, to be treated near his home or the home of his or her relatives or friends and shall have the right to return to the community as soon as possible.
3. Every patient shall have the right to treatment suited to his or her cultural background.

Principle 8: Standards of Care

1. Every patient shall have the right to receive such health and social care as is appropriate to his or her health needs and is entitled to care and treatment in accordance with the same standards as other ill persons.
2. Every patient shall be protected from harm, including unjustified medication, abuse by other patients, staff or other acts causing mental distress or physical discomfort.

Principle 9: Treatment

1. Every patient shall have the right to be treated in the least restrictive environment and with the least restrictive or intrusive treatment appropriate to the patient's health needs and the need to protect the physical safety of others.
2. The treatment and care of every patient shall be based on an individually prescribed plan, discussed with the patient, reviewed regularly, revised as necessary and provided by qualified staff.
3. Mental health care shall always be provided in accordance with applicable standards of ethics for mental health practitioners, including internationally accepted standards such as the Principles of Medical Ethics adopted by the United Nations General Assembly. Mental health knowledge shall never be abused.

4. The treatment of every patient shall be directed towards preserving and enhancing personal autonomy.

Principle 16: Involuntary Admission

1. A person may (a) be admitted involuntarily to a mental health facility as a patient; or (b) having already been admitted voluntarily as a patient, be retained as an involuntary patient in the mental health facility if, and only if, a qualified mental health practitioner authorised by law for that purpose determines, in accordance with Principle 4 [determination of mental illness], that a person has a mental illness and considers:

   (a) that because of that mental illness, there is a serious likelihood of immediate or imminent harm to that person or to other persons; or

   (b) that in the case of a person whose mental illness is severe and whose judgement is impaired, failure to admit or retain that person is likely to lead to a serious deterioration in his or her condition or will prevent the giving of appropriate treatment that can only be given by admission to a mental health facility in accordance with the principle of least restrictive alternative.

   In the case referred to in subparagraph (b), a second such mental health practitioner, independent of the first, should be consulted where possible. If such consultation takes place, involuntary admission or retention may not take place unless the second mental health practitioner concurs.

Principle 17: Review Body

1. The review body shall be a judicial or other independent and impartial body established by domestic law and functioning in accordance with procedures laid down by domestic law. It shall, in formulating its decisions, have the assistance of one or more qualified and independent mental health practitioners and take their advice into account.
2. The review body's initial review . . . of a decision to admit or retain a person as an involuntary patient shall take place as soon as possible after that decision. . . .
6. If at any time the mental health practitioner responsible for the case is satisfied that the conditions for retention of a person as an involuntary patient are no longer satisfied, he or she shall order the discharge of that person as such a patient.

Principle 18 – Procedural Safeguards

1. The patient shall be entitled to choose and appoint a counsel to represent the patient as such, including representation in any complaint, procedure or appeal. If the patient does not secure such services, a counsel shall be made available without payment by the patient to the extent that the patient lacks sufficient means to pay.
2. The patient shall also be entitled to the assistance if necessary, of the services of an interpreter. Where such services are necessary and the patient does not secure them, they shall be made available without payment by the patient and to the extent that the patient lacks sufficient means to pay.

Legislators and policy-makers may also find it helpful to refer to the following World Health Organisation documents:

- *Guidelines for the Promotion of Human Rights of Persons with Mental Disorders*
- *Mental Health Care Law: Ten Basic Principles*

DETERMINING THE SCOPE AND OBJECTIVES OF MENTAL HEALTH LEGISLATION

Compliance with the rights and freedoms set out in the International Bill of Human Rights and other relevant human rights instruments will be a major factor in determining the scope of mental health legislation. However, as mentioned above, mental health and related legislation must support the mental health strategy.

Thus the development of mental health legislation must accord with the overall mental health strategy and assist in its implementation. The first step in this process will be to establish agreed principles upon which the legislation should be based, taking into account the need to protect human rights and the overall aims of the mental health strategy.

Examples of some suggested general principles, which are intended broadly to reflect the UN Principles, are set out below:

1. Respect for individuals and their social, cultural, ethnic, religious and philosophical values.
2. Individuals' needs taken fully into account.
3. Care and treatment provided in the least restrictive environment compatible with the care and safety of the individual and the safety of the family and the public.
4. Provision of care and treatment aimed at promoting each individual's self-determination and personal responsibility.
5. Provision of care and treatment aimed at achieving the individual's own highest attainable level of health and well-being.

Agreeing on the general principles will assist the legislators in determining the aims and objectives of the legislation and defining the scope of the statutory powers, duties and rights. This can be demonstrated by looking at the five suggested principles in further detail.

1. Respect for individuals and their social, cultural, ethnic, religious and philosophical values

This embraces the other general principles and may be the most difficult to frame within legislation. However legislation could underpin this principle in the following ways:

- Outlaw unfair discrimination, making it unlawful to treat a person less favourably than others on the grounds of the person's disability (mental illness could be included in the definition of disability or treated as a separate category), race, sex, religion or other status where such a distinction is not justified. Such anti-discrimination legislation would probably be separate to mental health legislation.
- Establish monitoring and evaluation mechanisms to ensure that the standards of mental health care are of the same level as the care provided to people with physical health needs.
- The provision of interpreters – providing all people who have difficulties in communicating and are being assessed for, or receiving, mental health services, with access to an independent, properly trained interpreter.
- Establish an accessible complaints procedure – providing all people receiving mental health services with the right to pursue any complaints they may have about the services provided. It would not be necessary for mental health legislation to cover this area; it may be more appropriate to have separate legislation dealing with complaints procedures for the relevant bodies, such as health and social care agencies.
- The provision of advocacy services. States may also wish to consider developing services which enable those who are subject to, or being assessed for, compulsory detention and/or treatment, to have access to an independent, properly trained advocate. Any such advocates would be separate and additional to the legal representatives available, in accordance with UN Principle 18(1) (see page 48), to individuals detained under mental health legislation.

The implementation of such provisions would need to be supported by other parts of the strategy, such as providing accessible information to service users and their family and friends caring for them ('carers'), training staff and developing equal opportunities policies within health and social care agencies.

2. Individuals' needs taken fully into account

The principle that individuals' needs should be taken fully into account is closely connected to the first and third principles. It also flows from the identification of the 'seven irreducible elements of care' (discussed in Chapter 8 below) such as accommodation and social support, which people with mental illness are likely to need and the corresponding aim to develop comprehensive mental health services.

To ensure that individuals have access to these elements of care, legislation should provide for:

- the comprehensive assessment of individuals' needs for health care (mental and physical), social care and other types of support, such as housing;
- the assessment procedure to include the requirement to seek and take into account individuals' views and wishes.

Such an assessment should extend beyond mental health care and will require close liaison between health, social care and other care agencies. Thus, mental health legislation should facilitate effective joint working across these agencies.

3. Care and treatment provided in the least restrictive environment compatible with the care and safety of the individual and the safety of the family and the public

This principle reflects the generally accepted view that, as far as possible, individuals should have the opportunity of being cared for and treated in the community in which they live.

In order to uphold this principle, which is linked to the rights to liberty and private and family life, mental health legislation should be framed so that compulsory hospital admission is a last resort and lasts no longer than necessary. Thus legislation must ensure that an individual is only detained where:

- there are clearly defined grounds for detention;
- the lawfulness of the detention is open to independent review;
- procedural safeguards are in place.

(a) *There are clearly defined grounds for detention*

Case-law under the European Convention of Human Rights has established that (except in emergencies) the following conditions must be met to justify detention on the grounds of mental disorder (Winterwerp v. The Netherlands (1979)):

- The person must be reliably shown to be of 'unsound mind' – objective medical opinion must establish a true mental disorder.
- The mental disorder must be of a kind or degree warranting compulsory confinement.
- The validity of continued detention depends on the persistency of such a mental disorder.

(b) *The lawfulness of the detention is open*
to independent review

Ensuring that there is an independent review of the decision to detain an individual is a crucial safeguard for those who have been detained, and should require:

- all members of the review body to be independent of the State and the parties to the case;
- the provision of training for members of the review body on their role;
- access to independent medical opinion;
- that the review takes place as soon as possible after the detention has been initiated;
- if detention continues, a periodic review at reasonable intervals;
- the review panel to have the power to order the individual's release if the grounds for detention are no longer met.

(c) *Procedural safeguards are in place*

In addition to the independent review, these safeguards would include:

- information about the review process and other rights under the legislation;
- access to legal advice and representation;
- access to an interpreter if required;
- the decision of the review panel to be in writing.

4. Provision of care and treatment aimed at promoting each individual's self-determination and personal responsibility

It is vital that individuals are given the opportunity to exercise choice and make decisions about their own care and treatment. Legislation should aim to ensure that:

- treatment and care are provided to meet the assessed needs of each individual;
- treatment can be given without consent only in strictly limited circumstances and must be the least restrictive and invasive alternative;
- where individuals are unable to make decisions about their treatment, procedures must ensure that treatment is only given in their best interests and steps are taken to find out their wishes and feelings;
- clear information on treatment and detention is readily available;
- patient confidentiality is protected.

5. Provision of care and treatment aimed at achieving the individual's own highest attainable level of health and well-being

This principle covers issues such as quality and continuity of care, in addition to the need to ensure that individuals should be cared for properly in a safe environment and that restrictions on individuals' rights and freedoms are kept to an absolute minimum. In this regard mental health legislation should:

- ensure that there are no restrictions on an individual's contact with friends and family, save for exceptional and clearly defined circumstances;
- provide stringent safeguards from abuse exploitation and neglect;
- protect the civil rights of people with mental illness – for example, the fact of detention should not affect the person's right to vote or marry.

PUTTING PRINCIPLES AND RIGHTS INTO PRACTICE: ISSUES AND QUESTIONS

In order to ensure the effective implementation of mental health and related legislation it must be developed in consultation with users of mental health services, carers, professionals and other stakeholders. Thus the mental health strategy should include mechanisms which enable the views of interested parties to be sought and taken into account. Some of the major issues and questions that are likely to arise in such discussions are explored below.

1. The scope of the legislation: Who will be subject to mental health legislation?

In order to ensure that any powers of compulsion provided under mental health legislation are not used arbitrarily, it will be necessary to be clear as to who will fall within the scope of such powers. As discussed in Chapter 1, there are a variety of terms that are commonly used in relation to mental ill health. The following are examples of such terms which, if used to identify those who may subject to mental health legislation, must be defined in such legislation:

- Mental disorder
- Mental illness
- Psychopathic disorder
- Personality disorder
- Learning disabilities
- Mental impairment
- Acquired brain disorders.

The decision that an individual has a condition that falls within the scope of the legislation must be reached on an objective basis. This is made clear in Principle 4 of the United Nations Principles which state that the determination that a person has a mental illness must be based on 'internationally accepted standards'.

One example of an internationally accepted standard is the *International Statistical Classification of Diseases and Related Health Problems* (ICD-10). The draft *Mental Health Act of Zanzibar* (Ministry of Health, 1998) includes this in its definition of mental disorder:

> ' "Mental disorder" means a significant occurrence of a mental or behavioural disorder classified in the latest edition of the *International Classification of Diseases* published by the World Health Organisation.'

As discussed in Chapter 1, the terminology used in mental health may be controversial while there are different views of 'mental illness' and different local and regional explanations of this condition. This should be borne in mind when developing mental health legislation and is an issue on which it would be beneficial to hold discussions with professionals, service users and other stakeholders in order to gain a general consensus on acceptable terminology.

However, it is crucial that the legislation makes clear that an individual's values or beliefs should never be a factor in determining whether the person has a mental illness. Neither should socially deviant behaviour of itself determine mental illness. Mental illness may have social causes and social consequences, but this is not the same as social deviancy. (See also page 5.)

2. Respecting individuals' autonomy: The need to achieve a proper balance between protecting the rights of the individual and ensuring public safety

While ensuring that the rights and freedoms of individuals are respected, there may be occasions when it will be necessary to restrict the rights and freedoms of an individual in order to secure the rights and freedoms of others. This is acknowledged in Article 29(4) of the Universal Declaration:

> 'In the exercise of his rights and freedoms, everyone shall be subject to such limitations as are determined by law solely for the purpose of securing due recognition and respect for the rights and freedoms of others and of meeting the just requirements of morality, public order and the general welfare in a democratic society.'

The question of whether an individual's rights and freedoms should be restricted and, if so, in what circumstances will be a crucial consideration in the development of mental health legislation. The need to closely define the circumstances in which individuals may be detained on grounds of their mental disorder was discussed above in connection with UN Principle 4. Similar considerations will apply to treatment for mental disorder – it will be necessary to decide whether individuals may be treated for their mental disorder without their consent and, if so, in what circumstances. In deciding the scope of any compulsory treatment provisions in the mental health legislation, it may be helpful to consider the following points:

- The question of whether treatment may given without a person's consent arises in two situations:
  - (a) Where the individual does not have capacity to decide whether he or she wishes to receive treatment.
  - (b) Where the person has capacity to decide whether or not he or she wishes to receive, but refuses, the treatment proposed.

- Where the person lacks capacity to consent to treatment:
  - (a) Could treatment be provided in the person's 'best interests'?
  - (b) If so, how would 'best interests' be defined and who would be involved in determining what is in the person's best interests?

- Where the person has capacity to refuse the proposed treatment, in what circumstances can the individual's wishes be overridden?
  - (a) Where there is a risk of harm to others?
  - (b) Where there is a risk of harm to the individual? (For example, the person may try to commit suicide.)
  - (c) Where there is a risk to the health of the individual? (For example, the person's health may deteriorate.)

It will also be important to ensure that there is a clear definition of 'consent' and 'capacity' and to develop a workable test for determining whether a person has the capacity to consent to treatment. Other issues for consideration include, for example, the question of whether 'advance statements' (the previously expressed wishes of a person about particular forms of treatment) should be taken into account when that person has subsequently lost the capacity to make such treatment decisions.

3. What treatments may be given for mental disorder?

The UN Principles give guidance on this area and state, for example, that:

- only medication of known or demonstrated efficacy may be administered (special procedures apply to clinical trials).
- sterilisation shall never be carried out as a treatment for mental illness;

- psychosurgery and other intrusive and irreversible treatments shall only be given with informed consent and when an independent external body has satisfied itself that the patient has given informed consent and that the treatment best serves the health needs of the patient.

4. Dealing with emergencies

In drafting mental health legislation, consideration will need to be given to how to provide for circumstances in which immediate action is thought necessary and there is insufficient time to ensure compliance with the usual procedures.

Case-law under the European Convention acknowledges that in exceptional cases, for example in order to protect the public, an individual may be confined without first obtaining a medical opinion that he or she has a mental disorder. However, detention in such circumstances can be justified for only a short duration, and detention can only continue if the minimum conditions for detention, discussed above, have been met (X v. United Kingdom (1981)).

The UN Principles make it clear that physical restraint or the involuntary seclusion of individuals will only be justified in exceptional circumstances, stating that such actions shall not be employed except:

- in accordance with officially approved procedures of the mental health facility, and
- when this is the only means available to prevent immediate or imminent harm to the patient or others, and
- shall not be prolonged beyond the period in which they are strictly necessary.

5. Linking mental health services and the criminal justice system

The UN Principles highlight the need to ensure that prisoners who have or are believed to have a mental illness are provided with the best available mental health care. This will require access to appropriately qualified staff to assess and treat such individuals and the provision of suitable mental health care facilities. Legislation should set out the circumstances in which individuals can be admitted to mental health facilities and how this relates to decisions such as to whether a criminal investigation should be undertaken or, where the person has been convicted of an offence, if any sentence of imprisonment should be imposed.

6. Supporting carers of people with mental health problems

In many cases family and friends provide informal care and support to people with mental health problems. Mental health legislation should ensure a proper balance between enabling carers to receive sufficient assistance, so that they can continue to provide care and support, and ensuring that the rights of individuals with mental illness – for example, the right to privacy – are not undermined.

7. Other issues concerning legislation

In considering legislation to support the strategy, it is vital that an analysis of factors that are likely to affect its implementation is undertaken.

For example, if there is a shortage of doctors, legislation should take this into account when deciding who establishes whether the conditions for detention are met. The *Draft Mental Health Act of Zanzibar* (Ministry of Health, 1998) provides that a 'Health Officer' on duty in a mental health care setting is authorised (after carrying out a psychiatric examination) to decide whether an individual should be compulsorily admitted. The definition of 'Health Officer' is:

> 'A health care provider whose professional qualification is of the highest category among staff on duty at a mental health care setting, according to the following descending order of priority: medical doctors; psychiatric nurses; medical assistants.'

CHAPTER FIVE

Mental health information systems

By Dr Gyles Glover and the authors

Key Points

- *Action is needed nationally to develop integrated mental health information systems covering primary and secondary care.*
- *Such systems provide an essential resource for clinicians, managers, planners and policy-makers.*
- *Users and carers also require relevant information.*
- *All countries can develop comprehensive information strategies but the methods used for implementation will vary depending on resources and IT availability.*

OVERVIEW

The purpose of an information strategy is to provide each professional and patient (often via professionals but independently if wished/able) with the information they require to

- enable evidence-based or informed decision-making;
- access appropriate services;

and, for users and carers, the better information should:

- set out for them the choices they could make;
- establish them more as equal partners in their own care.

The aim is to strengthen both patient and professional in their own decision-making and in the way they can interact, leading to greater satisfaction and better outcomes from mental health care.

Good information is also essential to ensure effective planning, budgeting, delivery of mental health care, evaluation and documentation of the outcomes of resource expenditure. In addition, the public importance of national statistics and providing numerical evidence about matters of social significance is increasingly recognised. Ideally, an information framework should indicate the groups of people (e.g. by age, gender, ethnic group, social class) who are receiving care, their specific types of mental health problems, the care they are receiving, the results of that care, and how satisfied they are. While most service-oriented systems will be developed in specialist mental health services, it is important to recognise that they must also cover primary care and social care.

The strategy must ensure that adequate safeguards are in place to ensure that personal information about individual patients is treated as, and remains, confidential. The right to privacy and the right of individuals to the protection of the law against interference with their privacy is set out in Article 17 of the International Covenant of Civil and Political Rights. Principle 6 of the UN Principles for the Protection of Persons with Mental Illness states:

> *The right of confidentiality of information concerning all persons to whom the present Principles apply shall be respected.*

A total information strategy needs to provide for five distinct information streams:

1. Patient records and patient information. This should ideally integrate health (primary and secondary care) and social care.
2. Information on the evidence base. Traditionally this comes from libraries and journals, but is increasingly coming from the internet.
3. Consumer information that can be provided to patients. This often comes from NGOs in the form of leaflets, etc., but much of this information is now internet based.
4. Local service and access information.
5. A management stream of information which, as described above, extracts key data on service utilisation, epidemiology, etc., from the patient record system.

Ultimately, many countries will wish to move to an integrated IT-based system to provide all five information streams, making use of internet resources. However, it is important to emphasise that the basic information requirements of all five data streams can be met with paper-based systems or with limited IT capability. They depend more on design, organisation and management commitment than the amount of resource available to purchase IT. Inability to purchase hardware should not be an obstacle to developing a simple, but effective, information strategy.

KEY QUESTIONS TO BE ADDRESSED

Planning questions include:

- How many people are there in each administrative area with mental health problems who need treatment at primary care level? How many people are there who need treatment at secondary care level? What proportion are currently getting care at the appropriate level?
- Are the available staff and other resources distributed appropriately, with proportionately more in areas of greater need?
- Is there any evidence that the number needing care is changing?
- Are there sufficient safeguards to protect patient confidentiality?

Evaluation questions include:

- Are the primary and specialist services reaching the appropriate people?
- Does the spread of problems identified and treated, and the outcomes in each area, suggest that primary care and specialist care services are functioning well?
- Do the amounts and combinations of care given for the types of problem encountered vary between areas and do they appear to be an efficient use of resources?
- Where compulsory detention and treatment is used for mental illness, what numbers and types of people are affected, and for how long and in what ways?

Questions relevant to care delivery

- Administratively, what range of primary care and specialist care support and supplies is needed in each area?
- Clinically, where the care of individuals is shared and deputies cover non-working hours or holidays, staff will commonly need simple summary records of patients they are called upon to see. Questions will include: What problems have been identified in the past? Do they pose any risk to themselves or others? What treatment has been planned and is it happening?

BUILDING THE INFORMATION STRATEGY

From the 'Top Down' the first task is identifying the areas or community frameworks within which primary and specialist mental health care is delivered, and establishing the size and composition of their populations. Reference to research work combined with knowledge of local features such as migrant and refugee groups will then allow estimation of the likely numbers of people with problems requiring treatment.

From the 'Bottom Up', primary care and specialist care out-patient and in-patient units need to provide details of the numbers and types of staff available, the numbers of people treated, the nature of their problems, the care given and the outcomes.

In all countries the bulk of mental health care happens in primary care, and many poor countries have only very sparse specialist services. For both these reasons, mental health information in primary care is extremely important. In many African countries, there already exists a primary health care unit information form, known as the stroke form, which records the age, sex and diagnosis of every consultation in primary care. Unfortunately, the form only has one catch-all category for the whole of mental illness despite containing 34 categories for physical illness. This, of course, is no help at all for planning requirements for essential medicines, training needs, etc.

TECHNICAL ISSUES

Data handling

Technically, the simplest format for data returns is as a set of summary tables for each administrative area covering the issues discussed above, and tailored to reflect national needs, preoccupations and priorities. Where possible, the information required should be recorded in agreed forms, as part of the process of clinical care, in notes, which are locally useful for clinical communication. Where simple computing systems are available, the establishment of local case registers using simple and freely available systems, such as the WHO software package EPI-INFO, will permit easy extraction of statistical tables for both local and national use. Where resources for information technology are more extensive, networked systems supporting fully electronic patient notes are available.

Coding

Statistical analysis of information about mental health care requires data structured to permit simple tabulation. The nature and scope of problems at presentation and as they progress, and the interventions administered, require classification to permit analysis. In routine practice, as opposed to research, classifications such as the ICD are likely to prove too onerous. Where services are mainly primary care based, simple broad groupings including depression, anxiety, schizophrenia, bipolar disorder, dementia, substance abuse, intellectual disability, etc., may be used to establish treatment requirements. Scales to measure health outcomes specifically designed for use in routine clinical practice are beginning to emerge, e.g. HoNOS (Wing et al., 1996).

OTHER ELEMENTS OF THE STRATEGY

Evidence base

It may be worth inviting an individual or organisation to bring together the available evidence base into a national library for mental health – this can either be electronic if resources permit or hard copy. In either case imaginative alternative ways of getting the evidence base to professionals should be considered, such as bulletins, reviews, cascade methods, meetings, etc. Some of the evidence base is already accessible on the internet, so duplication should be avoided. Countries which cannot afford to give information technology to each individual clinician can consider equipping local centres with key information. Even a single desktop computer with a telephone link within a health facility could revolutionise access to information.

Consumer information

It may also be worth asking a respected NGO to bring together the best currently available consumer information and develop a strategy for ensuring that it is effectively disseminated via hard copy and IT. Even in wealthy countries most consumers will continue to want hard copy material or face-to-face discussion as the main methods of receiving information. In some cases carers will have different information requirements, and telephone helplines have been of great assistance in many countries.

Local services

Each administrative area should produce a simple directory of local mental health and other relevant services which should be available for clinicians and patients to consult in all relevant health facilities, libraries, etc.

Results of implementing information strategy

- Ability to direct government action and resources to areas where problems are currently most poorly addressed.
- Information to argue more cogently for the amounts and types of resources needed.
- Infrastructure to develop quality control mechanisms, permitting early identification of services under intolerable strain or failing to achieve appropriate outcomes.
- Better informed users and professionals.
- Improved clinical practice.
- Patient empowerment.

Consequences of inaction

- Little evidence to determine cost implications or rational introduction strategy for new and possibly expensive treatments.
- Lack of awareness of scale of national context makes it difficult to handle news stories about rare tragedies or serious incidents.
- Poor quality planning.
- Slower implementation of the evidence base.
- Poorly informed patients.

CHAPTER SIX

Mental health promotion

Key Points

- *Mental health promotion is a fundamental part of health promotion generally.*
- *The positive steps individuals can take to protect their own mental health are well understood.*
- *Certain settings are strategic priorities for mental health promotion, including the family, schools, the workplace and the local community.*
- *There is good evidence for the effectiveness of mental health promotion.*

Most countries have a range of initiatives in place to promote physical health – for example, strategies to reduce smoking, drug and alcohol misuse or to promote improved diet or safer sex. However, there is much less awareness of the importance of promoting mental health, of the value of addressing mental health as part of general health programmes and of the interrelationship between mental, physical and social well-being. Initiatives like World Mental Health Day, which is celebrated on 10 October each year, provide a valuable opportunity to highlight the global significance of mental health and to focus public attention on the importance of taking action to promote mental well-being, particularly for children and young people.[1]

In developing a mental health strategy, it is crucial to demonstrate the relationship between mental well-being and physical health, and the influence that mental health has on behavioural problems, violence, child abuse, drug and alcohol abuse, risk-taking behaviour (e.g. smoking and unsafe sex) and sickness absence in the workplace. Although treatment and prevention are important, a strategy which includes mental health promotion has a much wider range of social, economic and health benefits.

---

[1] World Mental Health Day was established by the World Federation for Mental Health and is co-sponsored by the World Health Organisation.

DEFINING MENTAL HEALTH PROMOTION

What is mental health promotion?

Mental health promotion can be seen as a kind of immunisation, working to increase the resilience of individuals, families, organisations and communities, as well as to reduce conditions which are known to damage mental well-being in everyone, whether or not they currently have a mental health problem (HEA, 1998a, 1999a).

The value of mental health promotion

A secure family life, feeling safe, being able to participate in society, access to meaningful employment, adequate housing and support during times of vulnerability all have a positive impact on mental well-being. Strengthening the mental health of individuals, families, organisations and communities not only reduces vulnerability to mental health problems but also (International Union for Health Promotion and Education, 1999):

- improves physical health
- increases productivity
- reduces sickness absence at work
- reduces child abuse
- reduces behavioural and learning problems
- reduces risk-taking behaviour.

Effective mental health promotion

A meta study by Bosma & Hosman (1990) found that mental health promotion is most effective when interventions involve the social networks of those targeted, operate at a range of different points and times and use a combination of methods (e.g. improving coping or life skills and developing social support).

Mental health promotion is most effective when it intervenes at a range of different times in the life cycle, e.g. infancy and adolescence, is integrated within different settings, e.g. in schools and in primary care and is planned at different levels, e.g. locally, regionally and nationally.

A strategic approach to mental health promotion should aim to include a balance of:

- Developing coping/life skills, e.g. parenting, communication, negotiation.

- Promoting social support and networks, e.g. tackling bullying, supporting bereaved families, facilitating self-help groups, increasing access to information and opportunities to participate.
- Addressing structural barriers to mental health in such areas as education, employment, housing and income policy.

Possible goals for mental health promotion include:

- An increase in emotional literacy (parenting, schools, relationships).
- Reductions in social isolation (employment, support for elderly, access to services, improved local democracy).
- An increase in organisations with a mental health promotion policy (schools, workplaces, hospitals, prisons).

Mental health promotion is most effective when information and support are available, and the messages reinforced, in a wide range of settings. For example, within the family, during pregnancy and early childhood, in schools, in the workplace, in primary care, in places of worship, in the provision of local services and within community settings.

Protective and risk factors for mental health

It is important not to adopt a fatalistic approach to mental illness, particularly to disorders associated with trauma and deprivation. Psychological and psycho-social variables – for example, levels of self-esteem and life skills, including communication, negotiation and conflict management – may have a significant influence on the impact of socio-economic factors and individual, family or community responses to trauma or stressful life events.

The impact of risk factors for mental health problems – e.g. bereavement, a family history of psychiatric disorders or unemployment – can be reduced by strengthening factors known to protect mental well-being. Many risk factors for mental health problems are difficult to address, notably those arising from political conflict, long-term economic problems or natural disasters. A strategic framework for mental health promotion therefore needs to achieve a balance between reducing risk factors and strengthening protective factors, which can enhance the ability of communities to cope with and survive difficulties.

Protective and risk factors for mental health can be identified at three levels: individual, community and structural. They can be addressed at different stages of life (e.g. childhood, old age), in different settings (e.g. school, workplace) and at different levels (e.g. within the family, regionally or nationally), as shown in Figure 6.1.

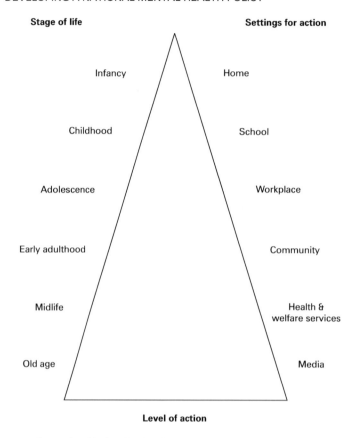

Stage of life

Infancy

Childhood

Adolescence

Early adulthood

Midlife

Old age

Settings for action

Home

School

Workplace

Community

Health &
welfare services

Media

Level of action

International/national/regional/local community/family/individual

FIG. 6.1

Risk/protective factors for individuals

Risk factors can be broadly defined as circumstances or experiences which reduce emotional resilience. These include:

- Physical illness or disability
- Low self-esteem and social status
- Feelings of helplessness
- Basic needs not being met, e.g. homelessness
- Separation and loss
- Violence or abuse
- Substance misuse
- Family history of psychiatric problems
- Childhood neglect.

Protective factors include:

- Physical health
- Positive sense of self
- Life/coping skills
- Basic needs are met
- Positive experience of early bonding
- Opportunities to learn.

Risk/protective factors for communities

Risk factors for communities are those which erode the capacity of communities to build strong social networks, to participate in community life, to have a say in decisions from higher levels in society which affect the life of the community and to access basic services. Such risk factors include:

- Cultural conflict
- Discrimination
- Inequality
- Unemployment
- Fear of violence
- Bullying.

Protective factors include:

- Strong social networks
- Positive role models
- Employment
- High levels of participation
- Opportunities to make choices, exercise control, develop skills
- Tolerance and trust.

Structural risk/protective factors for countries

The risk factors include:

- Poverty
- Inequality
- Unemployment
- Poor quality housing/physical environment
- Political conflict.

The protective factors include:

- Positive educational experiences – notably pre-school
- Safe, secure environment
- Peace.

The different levels of mental health promotion

There are three distinct levels of mental health promotion in order to address the risk/protective factors described above:

- Strengthening individuals or increasing emotional resilience through interventions designed to promote self-esteem, life and coping skills, communicating, negotiating, relationship and parenting skills; and skills to improve the capacity to cope with life events, transitions and stresses, e.g. parenting, bereavement, redundancy, unemployment, retirement.
- Strengthening communities, e.g. increasing social inclusion and participation, improving neighbourhood environments, developing health and social services which support mental health, anti-bullying strategies at school, child care schemes, workplace health, community safety, and supporting and facilitating social and self-help support networks.
- Reducing structural barriers to mental health through initiatives to reduce discrimination and inequality and to promote access to education, meaningful occupation, adequate housing, and appropriate services and support for those who are vulnerable, e.g. disabled or chronically ill, refugees, immigrants, prisoners.

A strategic approach to mental health promotion should aim to include a balance of developing coping skills (e.g. parenting, communication, promoting social support) and networks (e.g. tackling bullying, supporting bereaved families, facilitating self-help groups) and addressing structural barriers to mental health in such areas as education, employment and housing.

KNOWLEDGE, ATTITUDES AND AWARENESS ABOUT MENTAL HEALTH PROMOTION

Because mental illness is deeply tabooed, there is a consequent widespread lack of understanding and awareness of:

- how to look after mental health;
- how to recognise and act on early signs of mental distress;
- when to seek help; and
- types of help available.

A deeper understanding of mental health issues helps to reduce the stigma attached to seeking help and to assist people to seek help appropriately, as well as to increase awareness of simple self-help techniques for managing distress. Many people have a role in identifying early symptoms of mental disorder, including parents, teachers, spiritual leaders and community workers. Early identification and treatment, together with a greater understanding of the role of social support in prevention and mediating symptoms, are important factors in reducing the burden on primary care.

There is good evidence that the following 'positive steps' enhance mental well-being, facilitate coping with problems and enable people to deal with minor episodes of mental distress.

- Self-acceptance
- Physical activity
- Relaxation/stress management
- Reducing alcohol consumption to moderate levels
- Opportunities to talk about problems
- Opportunities to learn new skills
- Creative or spiritual activity, e.g. prayer, music
- Participation in community life
- Strong friendship/social networks
- Ability to seek help.

'Positive steps' for mental health can be promoted in a wide range of settings and services, including schools, workplaces, primary care units and within prisons, hospitals and other residential settings, as well as via public education campaigns like World Mental Health Day (Jenkins, 2001c).

Mental health promotion has a key role to play in reducing fear and anxiety about mental health problems and creating a climate of public opinion which acknowledges that people with mental health problems have a contribution to make. Stigma reinforces discrimination against people with mental health problems in important ways, notably in employment, and may also inhibit service delivery within the community. It also prevents people from seeking help and contributes centrally to the difficulties faced by people with mental health problems, their friends, families and carers.

STRATEGIC PRIORITIES FOR ACTION

Support for parents

There is strong evidence that the early years have a crucial impact on mental health throughout a person's life, and investment in the mental health of young children is therefore of fundamental importance. This involves raising awareness of the significance of the mental well-being of children, as well as interventions to support parenting, to facilitate positive relationships between parents and children, to improve child-rearing conditions and to protect vulnerable children. Early support during pregnancy for mothers in difficult social and economic circumstances has been shown to have a positive impact on birth weight as well as family relationships (Barker et al., 1992; Olds, 1998; Mental Health Europe, 1999 – www.mhe-sme.org/enmhp).

For this reason, all health workers will need to be aware of mental health promotion and the value of psycho-social support, which can be integrated with existing programmes for maintaining the physical health of mothers and infants, e.g. breastfeeding, immunisation, nutrition, weaning, etc. In a project in a township outside Cape Town, local, lay community workers were used to provide this support, since no health sector staff were available (Richter, 1994).

Mental health promotion in schools

There are many examples of the effectiveness of mental health promotion in schools, which is just as important as physical health education and should be routinely included as part of the curriculum. Mental health promotion focuses on increasing children's self-esteem, self-confidence and psycho-social skills and may be integrated with programmes concerned with smoking, drug and alcohol abuse, and sex education. Life skills education can be carried out as part of existing subjects, focusing on positive lessons for dealing with the demands and challenges of everyday life. All children need opportunities to succeed, to be valued and to contribute to the life of the family, school and wider community. Greater community awareness of the needs of children can be developed through a partnership approach to such issues as bullying and the emotional needs of vulnerable children, by involving parents, religious leaders, local businesses or community groups (Weare & Gray, 1995; Durlak, 1995). Teachers also need basic training and support in the early detection of mental disorders as well as learning difficulties like dyslexia, which, if untreated, greatly increase the risk of later problems.

The importance of opportunities to participate in, and perhaps influence, decisions which affect one's life has significant consequences for the design and delivery of services. Structures which facilitate community planning and local decision-making in the provision of services may have an impact on the health of the community in excess of the value of the services themselves. Mental health promotion has a crucial role to play in reducing and limiting the impact of psycho-social stressors, both through strengthening individuals, and through strengthening and supporting a diversity of social, communication and information networks, which link people within the community (Friedli, 1999).

Policy needs to ensure that the general health education programme – which is likely to have already established good links to schools, the media and health workers – now develops and includes education of the community about mental health and mental illness, about life skills and coping strategies, and about responsible community attitudes to people with a mental or physical disability. An example of such a school mental health programme has been evaluated in Pakistan (Rahman et al., 1998, Saeed et al., 1999).

Mental health promotion in the workplace

Employers are key stakeholders and there is a strong economic case for including mental health promotion in workplace health policies. Employers bear the cost of the consequences of untreated illness in terms of sickness absence, labour turnover, accidents and poor performance. Workplace policies should include information and support to enable workers with problems to get help, and should provide assistance for those recovering from mental health problems to re-enter the workplace (Jenkins & Warman, 1993). Employers can also take steps to promote mental health and thus reduce the risk of problems developing. Key risk factors for physical and mental health problems in the workplace are lack of control over the way work is organised and paced, high levels of uncertainty, poor communications and low levels of security and safety. Studies in the US, UK, Sweden and the Czech Republic have demonstrated a strong association between psycho-social factors at work and overall health, notably in relation to a risk of heart disease. It is therefore cost-effective for employers to place mental health promotion at the centre of their workplace health policies (Bobak et al., 1998; Johnson et al., 1996).

A number of studies in the UK have found that health service workers have greater levels of sickness absence and poorer mental health than those of employees generally, and this may be the case in other countries (Borrill et al., 1996).

There is also good evidence of the effectiveness of interventions with people who are unemployed, notably in reducing the risk of depression. Interventions with a strong focus on job search self-efficacy, social and emotional coping skills and building social support have been shown to be effective (Price et al., 1992).

Mental health promotion in the community

Mental health promotion in the community extends beyond initiatives to reduce stigma and projects within the specific settings of schools, workplaces or health centres. There is evidence that the strength of community life, high levels of social support, participation in social networks and opportunities for the exchange of skills and information, tend to reduce an individual's vulnerability to the mental and physical ill-effects of socio-economic stressors (Cooper et al., 1999). Initiatives to improve the environment, access to transport, community safety or rebuilding communities that have been damaged by political conflict or natural disaster are significant elements of an overall mental health strategy (HEA, 1998a). Recent epidemiological research has demonstrated a correlation between low levels of social trust and higher rates of most major causes of death, including coronary heart disease, maligant neo-plasms, strokes, accidents and infant mortality (Kawachi, 1997b).

Strengthening the mental well-being of communities

Few examples of community-wide interventions have been evaluated. There is, however, evidence that communities with low levels of trust, tolerance and opportunities for participation in decision-making have poorer physical and mental health, even when poverty levels are controlled for. A cross-sectional ecologic study based on data from 39 States in the USA found that lower levels of social trust were associated with higher rates of most major causes of death, including coronary heart disease, malignant neoplasms, cerebrovascular disease, unintentional injury and suicide.

Community-wide interventions which combine support for parents, access to voluntary groups and school programmes focusing on reducing bullying and increasing personal skills have been effective in reducing substance abuse and juvenile crime and aggression.

Support networks/self-help

There is considerable evidence that good personal support networks – for example, friendship or a confiding relationship – protect mental health and enable people to recover from stressful life events such as bereavement or financial problems (Whelan, 1993).

Mental health promotion has a crucial role to play in reducing and limiting the impact of psycho-social stressors, both through strengthening individuals and through strengthening and supporting a diversity of social, communication and information networks. These include self-help, advocacy, neighbourhood and voluntary activities, as well as structures which facilitate community planning and local decision-making in the provision of services (Bloom et al., 1985).

Self-help support, e.g. basic psycho-social information, relaxation advice plus referral for self-help or to a self-help group, is as effective as cognitive therapy and medication in treating generalised anxiety disorders (Cuijpers, 1997). Active participation in user groups also has a wide range of benefits (Barnes & Shardlow, 1997). A study in Munich of self-help initiatives found that the value of self-help support was worth more than £15 million per annum (Stark, 1998).

Reducing stigma/changing attitudes

Campaigns or mass media interventions, particularly if supported by local community action, can have a measurable impact on knowledge, attitudes and behavioural intentions. Campaigns which focus on advocacy techniques – for example generating unpaid publicity in the press, or setting the news agenda through creating positive mental health stories – can also play a proven role in influencing opinion formers and the climate of public opinion (Wolf et al., 1999).

Reducing risk of depression for unemployed

Group cognitive behavioural therapy has been shown to be effective in improving the mental health and employment outcomes in unemployed adults (Caplan et al., 1997; Vinokur et al., 1995; Vinokur & Ryn, 1991). Interventions with a strong focus on job search, self-efficacy, social and emotional coping skills and building social support are also effective (Price et al., 1992). It is realised that not all unemployed people are at equal risk of depression, but this kind of intervention could be replicated through job centres as this approach also focuses on finding pleasant activities and improving social networks. A number of studies have demonstrated the value of social support in mitigating the impact of stressful life events, including unemployment (Whelan, 1993; Rosengren, 1993).

Reducing alcohol consumption

A brief (10–15 minute) intervention from GP/primary care is effective in reducing alcohol consumption (NHS Centre for Reviews and Dissemination, 1997), and brief advice has resulted in a reduction of alcohol consumption of 25–35% and a reduction of 45% in a proportion of excessive drinkers (Ashenden et al., 1997). It has been suggested that routine or opportunistic screening for alcohol problems in A&E departments should be followed by a brief intervention (Peters et al., 1998).

Exercise

Evaluation of Balance for Life in Essex found that their ten-week programme of exercise significantly reduced depression and anxiety, and increased the overall quality of life and self-efficacy for exercise.

Sixty-eight per cent of clinically depressed patients had depression scores that became non-clinical within 3 months (Darbishire & Glenister, 1998).

Arts and creativity

In a review of 60 community-based arts projects, Matarasso found that participation in these projects brought a wide range of social benefits, including increased confidence, community empowerment, self-determination, improved local image and identity and greater social cohesion (Matarasso, 1997).

Arts on Prescription provides access to art and creative activities, including poetry, painting, music and pottery. Arts on Prescription can be combined with Prescription for Leisure, allowing entry to a range of activities for people experiencing mild to moderate depression. There is some evidence that arts activity for former psychiatric in-patients results in fewer re-admissions (Colgan et al., 1997; Brown, 1997; Philips & Robertson, 1996). Evaluation of the Arts on Prescription project in Stockport showed an improvement in GHQ scores, better self-concept, an increase in social activities and less use of other services (Huxley, 1997). In addition, the King's Fund has developed an evaluation framework suitable for arts-based health work, which was pioneered in partnership with 'Looking Well', an arts-based community project in North Yorkshire (Angus & Murray, 1996; Wynne-Owen, 1998).

The mental health impact of health services

Price (1998) suggests a strong case for a primary care led audit of current medical care practices to identify treatment policies and practices that may produce adverse mental health effects. This could be extended to include those aspects of service provision which create stress and could be linked to user consultation. Enhancing perceived personal control is a model that has evaluated positively (Taylor et al., 1997; Price, 1998).

Reducing stress

Large-scale stress workshops were used as part of a Healthy Cities Programme in Birmingham. The workshops covered the physical, cognitive and behavioural aspects of anxiety and stress and offered a wide range of options for managing stress. In a three-month follow-up, participants were less anxious, less distressed and more able to cope than those in control and placebo groups. The workshops, open to anyone, were successful in reaching and helping those whose problems were not detected in primary care (Brown & Cochrane, 1999).

Reducing marital breakdown

Modifying known risk factors for relationship problems, notably poor communications and problem-solving skills, was found to reduce marital break-up in participants at four- and five-year follow-up (Markman et al., 1988). The key emphasis was on modifying known risk factors for relationship problems, notably poor communications and problem-solving skills (Bloom et al., 1985).

Reducing social disorder, criminal behaviour, anxiety, depression and suicidal behaviour in young adults

The Olweus study showed that being a bully or a victim of bullying is a predictor for later problems, including conduct disorders, crime, alcohol abuse (bullies) and depression, anxiety and suicidal behaviour (victims). There is therefore a strong case for including the basics of the Olweus anti-bullying strategy as a key intervention for assisting the transition to adulthood. These include zero tolerance for bullying (every child has a right to be safe at school), a period of consultation and training which enables parents, teachers, school governors and the wider community to sign up to the principles of anti-bullying, and clearly understood strategies for reporting and acting on bullying incidents (Olweus, 1993).

Pre-school education can substantially decrease the chances of drug abuse 20 years later and interventions for children with behavioural problems can reduce the likelihood of developmental difficulties (Zoritch et al., 2000).

Respite care

Programmes which provide respite for carers of people who are highly dependent are effective in reducing stress, as are some psycho-social interventions which aim to enhance access to support and coping skills.

Reducing physical health problems

Poor mental health is a risk factor for many physical health problems and emotional distress makes people more vulnerable to physical illness.

- Depression increases the risk of heart disease four-fold, even when other risk factors like smoking are controlled for (Hippisley-Cox et al., 1998).
- Lack of control at work is associated with increased risk of cardiovascular disease (Bosma et al., 1997).

- Sustained stress or trauma increases susceptibility to viral infection and physical illness by damaging the immune system (Marmot et al., 1991; Stewart-Brown, 1998; Bloom et al., 1985).

FAITH COMMUNITIES AND MENTAL HEALTH

A growing number of studies emphasise the importance of religious beliefs to people with mental health problems: a high value is placed on support from religious communities and prayer, worship, belief, faith, reading scriptures and belonging to a religious community are significant factors.

And yet, within public health circles, religion is often seen as an adversary. Certainly service users report that strong faith is sometimes seen as a symptom of illness by mental health professionals. Of course rational science has a long history of opposing theology and current scepticism about spirituality is rooted in Enlightenment conflicts between science and the Church. And yet this same rational science is today producing evidence that the rigid distinction between mind and body is not as stable as we previously thought. There is increasing evidence that mental health has a profound effect on physical health. Nevertheless, there is considerable resistance in some quarters to the idea that spirituality can have an impact beyond those elements of religious experience that can be measured in randomised controlled trials.

In practice, where religious faith is acknowledged, it is often in limited terms – for example, in relation to diet or cultural practices surrounding bereavement. It is often regarded as important for ethnic minority groups, but an emphasis on race may obscure the importance of religious belief as a vital part of a person's sense of identity and community. Muslim or Jewish faith, for example, may be more important to someone's identity than their ethnic origin.

There is also a broader issue: for many people, religion is no longer the means of expression of spirituality, there is a need to recognise/ acknowledge a 'whatever it is in people' as part of our broader response to addressing health needs, and public health and mental health services have not engaged these issues very effectively.

On the other hand, we need to be careful not to set up an uncritical opposition between 'faith communities good' and 'mental health services bad'. The rejection and fear of people with mental health problems has been commonplace in many religions. Some religious groups describe mental health problems in ways which many mental health service users find alienating. Terms like 'sufferer' and 'afflicted', which are widely used within all faiths to convey the distressing nature of some symptoms of mental illnesses, can also make service users feel like victims.

The rejection of victim status and the reinterpretation of mental illness as a 'disease of meaning' has gained strong currency through the user/survivor movement. In this analysis, experiencing and coping with depression, hearing voices, visions or radical changes in thoughts and feelings can be frightening and distressing, but can also enrich people's lives. These examples of ambivalence remain to the extent that there is no clear-cut line or easy distinction to be made between some forms of religious inspiration and symptoms of psychosis. Visions, speaking in tongues and hearing voices may be interpreted as powerful expressions of faith and spirituality.

In fact, there are significant parallels in the concerns of faith communities and the user/survivor movement. These centre on the extent to which health professionals are equipped to engage with alternative conceptual frameworks for understanding, treating and managing mental health problems – whether such alternatives derive from secular, or spiritual, beliefs regarding mental health.

In spite of this unease, there are a number of developments in public health which are prompting a renewed interest in the relationship between religion and health and suggest that the nature of faith and its consequences for mental well-being are important issues for mental health promotion. Social inclusion, identified by the International Labour Organisation as a crucial strategy for tackling poverty world wide, has been adopted as a cross-cutting theme by a number of governments, and has been identified as fundamental to reducing inequalities – again underlining an important area in which faith communities can contribute.

While there are anecdotal accounts of the pathological effects of religion, reviews of the research literature have consistently found that religious involvement is associated with positive mental health outcomes (Ellison and Levin, 1998). Nevertheless, there are fears that spiritual or religious explanations for someone's behaviour may mean they do not get appropriate professional help when it is needed. Underpinning such concerns is an ongoing debate about appropriate treatment for mental health problems and who is, or should be, responsible for care and treatment. Many people with mental health problems have found great support within their congregation and have found prayer, worship, religious belief and belonging to a religious community both helpful and affirming. Equally, some people have been damaged by their experiences with religious groups. Religious explanations for mental health problems which blame individuals or look for sins in their lives to account for their problems can cause great suffering. This is, of course, equally true of some people's experiences with mental health services and a range of treatment regimes, including medication and ECT, and is reflected in the growing interest in alternative and complementary approaches to the management of mental health problems.

In this respect, and in relation to mental health problems, faith communities offer a forum for exploring issues which are at the heart of the search for a spiritual context and contemporary debates about meaning, identity, relationships and the role of religion in the twenty-first century. This entails moving beyond the view that the mosque, church or synagogue is simply an extension of the 'care package'.

Places of worship are also important settings for promoting the mental well-being of the whole community, as well as creating an environment in which people with mental health problems can feel involved, included and valued. Such a shift in emphasis – from faith communities as service providers for people with mental health problems, to faith communities as mental health promoters – has great potential.

Many religious people have experienced mental health problems and some have expressed the impact of this on their faith. Recognition of how common such mental health problems are, and the extent of the shared experience of mental distress within a congregation, can provide a strong foundation from which to explore the meaning and value of mental health promotion within the expression of religious faith. From this perspective, faith communities have an important role to increase understanding of mental health issues and challenge stigma and discrimination – e.g. by combining new approaches to mental health with a long tradition, within churches, synagogues and mosques, of advocacy for local people, both individuals and communities.

In increasing understanding of the significance of mental health to all health and well-being, and in tackling factors which erode mental health – notably inequality and social exclusion – faith communities have powerful potential as allies for mental health promotion. However, it will require goodwill, lateral thinking and some leaps of the imagination to form the partnerships necessary to make the most of this opportunity – and to link it to a renewed engagement with spirituality as expressed both within and without formal religion.

CHAPTER SEVEN

Primary care

Key Points

- *Primary health care has a fundamental role to play in the mental health strategy – specialist services will only ever be able to deal with a small proportion of disorders.*
- *A range of issues concerning the efficient and effective working of primary care in tackling mental health are identified.*
- *The policy issues needing to be tackled to support primary care are identified, of which professional training is key.*

Primary health care has been defined by the World Health Organisation as:

> essential health care made accessible to individuals and families in the community by means acceptable to them, through their full participation and at a cost that the community and the country can afford. It forms an integral part of the country's health system of which it is the nucleus and of the overall social and economic development of the community. (WHO, 1978)

THE IMPORTANCE OF PRIMARY CARE
TO THE MENTAL HEALTH STRATEGY

The need for a strategy for mental health in primary care stems from the burden of the disorders in primary care, their cost to society, the actual and potential availability of specialist care and the unique positioning of the primary care team.

Mental disorder is extremely common

Mental disorder is extremely common in all countries in all parts of the world and no country can afford sufficient specialists to look after everyone with a mental disorder. Most people with a mental disorder, whoever they are and whatever the disorder, will need to be seen in primary care. The high prevalence (Shepherd et al., 1966; Harding et al., 1980; Regier et al., 1978; Goldberg & Huxley, 1992; Ustun & Sartorius, 1995), severity, duration (Mann et al., 1981) and accompanying disability (Jenkins et al., 1998) of mental health problems at the level of primary care has major implications.

The sheer volume of disorders means that it can never be remotely viable to plan to tackle them by exclusive use of specialist care. This is because even in relatively rich nations, specialist care can only usually cater for around 10% of the total number of people with mental health problems, and these will of necessity tend to be those with the greatest needs.

The need to recognise the burden of common mental disorders

It is no longer tenable to argue that the burden of common mental disorders can be ignored – the costs of doing so are immense in terms of repeated GP consultations (Lloyd et al., 1996), sickness absence (Jenkins, 1985b), labour turnover (Jenkins, 1985c), reduced productivity, impact on families and children. In addition there is the more difficult to quantify, but nonetheless important concept of the emotional well-being of a country and nation which undoubtedly influences its future.

Undetected and untreated morbidity in primary care

There is a significant amount of undetected morbidity and much untreated morbidity in primary care. A major WHO collaborating study in 15 primary care sites in developed and low-income countries round the world (Ustun and Sartorius, 1995) found:

- overall, primary care physicians identify 23.4% of the attenders as being a 'case' with a psychological disorder, while an interview using a research instrument identifies 33%;
- the primary physicians reported that they provided treatment to 77.8% of the cases whom they identified as having a psychological disorder (around half are given counselling, a quarter sedative medication and only one sixth receive antidepressants).

The primary care aspect of the mental health strategy needs to pay attention to planning at government level (e.g. ministers of health, education, social welfare, finance, etc.), at district level in terms of commissioning of services, and at local level. It is important to consider the various levers for change that might exist, e.g. legislation governing primary care activity, contracts of employment, commissioning of the work of the primary care team, training, the skill mix in a primary care team, and their continuing education.

INTERNATIONAL MOVES TOWARDS INTEGRATION OF MENTAL HEALTH IN PRIMARY CARE

Given the burden of common mental health problems, the integration of mental health with primary care services has been a significant policy objective in wealthy and low-income areas of the world (Lambo, 1996; Shepherd, 1980; Burns et al., 1979; Jenkins, 1992). Different countries are at varying stages of putting in place mechanisms for integrating mental health care into the work of primary care teams. Some of the most well-developed and proactive examples are to be found in low-income countries where the organisation has often been closely influenced by WHO and has followed a public health model (Schulsinger & Jablensky, 1991; Kilonzo & Simmons, 1998; Joop de Jong, 1996).

WHO (1984) has identified the crucial aspects for the successful design and implementation of a primary mental health care programme, which includes:

- Formulation of a national policy on mental health and the establishment of a mental health department or unit within each country's national or regional government.
- Financial provision for
  - the recruitment and training and employment of personnel
  - the adequate supply of essential medicines
  - a network of facilities including transport
  - data collection and research.
- Decentralisation of mental health services, integration of mental health services with the general health services, and the development of collaboration with non-medical community agencies.
- Use of non-specialised mental health workers including primary health workers, nurses, medical assistants and doctors, for certain basic tasks of mental health care.
- Training of mental health professionals in this new task of training and supporting non-specialised health workers.

Other significant international and UN agencies are starting to acknowledge the importance of tackling mental health issues if they are to achieve their broader goals. Despite this acknowledgement, it is important to recognise that in all countries physical illnesses are given a higher priority than mental illnesses, and there is a common view that primary care should not dilute its efforts for tackling physical illness by taking on the extra burden of mental disorders. However, there are several strong reasons to show why the integration of mental health into primary care is essential:

- *To achieve good clinical and social outcomes*   To obtain good care for people with a mental disorder who may not be able to see a specialist. In relatively rich countries this includes the majority of people with a common disorder such as depression and anxiety, while most if not everyone with a psychotic illness would expect to be able to see a specialist. In low-income countries where there may not be a specialist within hundreds of miles, it will also include most people with psychosis.
- *To ensure that physical health care needs are not neglected*   Physical and mental illness frequently co-exist and so exclusive preoccupation with a single speciality may be disastrous for the individual patient. People with severe mental illness have relatively high-standardised mortality ratios from physical ailments such as cardiac disease, respiratory disease, malignancy and, in low-income countries, infectious diseases. (Harris & Barraclough, 1998, *see also* p. 134.)
- *To address accompanying social needs*   Many psychiatric disorders are connected with family problems and social difficulties, and are only understandable when viewed against this background. Primary care teams with their continuing contact with their local population are well placed to have such detailed knowledge. The co-location of social workers with or working in association with primary health care teams may be helpful in delivering integrated health and social care.
- *To provide continuity of care*   Primary care teams are well placed to provide long-term follow-up and support without frequent changes of personnel.
- *To take account of the patient's perspective*   Many people with mental disorders do not consider themselves to be in need of psychiatric care and there may be less stigma for the patient if seen in primary care.

The challenge for primary care

Having emphasised the vast scale of the problem, the advantages of the primary care setting, and the scope for prevention in primary care, how can the busy primary care team possibly deliver in the midst of all the other competing obligations?

IMPLICATIONS OF MENTAL DISORDERS
IN PRIMARY CARE

Implications for national mental health policies

National mental health policies historically have tended to allow the specialist services to focus on the care of people with severe mental illness, and particularly on the care of mentally disordered offenders, but have tended to ignore the care of people with less severe disorders in primary care. They have also ignored the role of primary care in relation to the physical health care of severe mental illness. Such an approach is highly flawed because the lack of attention to the common mental disorders (which, if not adequately treated, greatly increase the burden to health services) will always compromise the care that can be targeted on people with severe mental illness, as well as cause immense costs for society. It is essential, therefore, that government policy should cover the whole spectrum of mental disorders so that the jigsaw puzzle of available services and disorders can articulate as a coherent whole.

Mental health policy at government level needs explicitly to address how the common mental disorders are to be tackled, who is responsible for their assessment, diagnosis and management, how quality standards for service inputs, processes and outcomes will be monitored; and the implications for human resources development, both basic training and continuing education.

Some contextual factors to be assessed before developing policy on primary care

Each country has its own unique health care delivery system and what makes sense in one country may not make sense in another. In the development of policy on primary–secondary care integration it is important to examine the existing primary and secondary care systems, staffing, basic and continuing training for each of the professional groups involved, and the system of information collection. While it is outside the scope of this review to provide a comprehensive account of the different organisational models of health care delivery, financing and coverage, the different degrees of provision of specialist care, the degree to which it has moved from a hospital-based system to a community system, and the role of primary care in each country, they are nonetheless important contextual factors for primary care integration and will be referred to from time to time. These issues are discussed below.

Does primary care perform a gatekeeping role?

In many low-income and certain Western countries, primary care performs an important gatekeeping function for secondary care, so that most consultations happen in primary care and only a relatively small proportion of people are subsequently referred to specialist care (Jenkins & Strathdee, 2000).

What is the composition of the primary care team?

This varies from country to country. In the UK, the primary care team consists of the general practitioner, practice manager, the practice nurse, possibly a counsellor, and linked community nurses such as health visitors and district nurses. In the USA the primary care worker may include the family doctor, the internist or even the gynaecologist or the paediatrician. In low-income countries, primary care may contain no doctors, possibly a few medical assistants, and be largely staffed by nurses and health workers with brief periods of training.

Who is in the front line?

Are the primary care doctor and nurse in the front line of assessment and treatment or is there another tier in the front line? For example, in some countries health workers with months rather than years of training are in the front line, dealing with screening and case finding, assessment and treatment, for a population of around 2,000 and they refer if necessary to the primary care doctor or nurse who may look after a population of 10,000. In Iran, the first tier is the village health worker; there is usually one male and one female for a population of 2,000.

Who is the lead professional in the primary care team?

Is the lead professional in the primary care team a doctor, or a medical assistant or a nurse, and what are their respective roles? In Zanzibar, the first tier is the primary health care unit which usually contains a medical assistant, and several male and female nurses. In Tanzania, the front line is the first aid volunteer, perhaps looking after 50 people; the second tier is the dispensary looking after 2,000 people; and the third tier is the primary health care unit run by nurses and medical assistants. In Pakistan, the first tier are health workers, usually married women with grown-up children, who receive a short training, and the second tier is the primary care doctor. In the UK the first tier, generally speaking, is the primary care doctor. Some still work alone but now most work in groups or partnerships of three to five and employ one or two primary care nurses between them. They also collaborate with a community nursing structure of district nurses and health visitors who are specialist nurses for older people and for young mothers with pre-school children, respectively.

Basic training of the primary care team

What does the basic training for each tier and professional in the primary care unit consist of and how much, if any, mental health training is included? In Iran, the health workers receive several months' training in a few priority topics which include reproductive health, infectious diseases, TB, schizophrenia and the common mental disorders such as depression and anxiety (Mohit, 1998). Addiction has recently been added to this list. The health workers are taught to screen and case-find by routine visits to homes, and to perform basic assessments, diagnoses and treatments in those conditions using good practice guidelines. They follow agreed criteria for referral to the primary care nurse and doctor who form the second tier of care, looking after a population of 10,000. In Zanzibar, the College of Health Sciences runs a four-year basic nursing course, of which the fourth year for women is midwifery and the fourth year for men is psychiatry. (The College has recently decided to add some psychiatry to the midwifery course.) A similar situation exists in Tanzania, and both countries now have a substantial population of primary care nurses who have received basic training in psychiatry.

Continuing education for the primary care team

What continuing training is available for each tier? In Zanzibar, there are education co-ordinators whose task is to organise and deliver continuing education for all the staff in the primary health care units. This continuing education is regular, consisting of several weekends a year for which the primary care staff receive transport allowances and incentive payments to attend. How much mental health is included in the regular continuing education? In most countries the continuing education programmes focus largely on physical illness and any mental health continuing education is an optional extra rather than an integrated component received by everyone.

Quality standards

What quality monitoring of standards in primary care exists? In Iran, health psychologists perform a quality-monitoring role for the health workers, visiting every month to support and supervise and check on the quality of the work.

Systems for information collection in primary care

Adequate planning is not possible without good systems for information collection in primary care. In Iran the health workers routinely collect basic data every year on the prevalence and outcome of the priority disorders which include infectious diseases, schizophrenia, epilepsy, depression and anxiety. This data is summarised into an annual table and displayed on the wall of the health centre. It is readily available to all staff who have the data and its implications for their work at their fingertips, and can be compared with preceding years. In some low-income countries, a stroke form is used for collecting consultation data in primary care, but while it contains 34 categories for separate physical disorders, it only contains one all-inclusive category for mental disorder.

Proactive approach

How proactive or reactive is the work of the primary care team? Does the primary care team mostly concentrate its time on those individual patients who actively consult, or does it take a more population-based approach and seek to find and treat the common disabling conditions in that population?

Capacity for outreach

In many countries, especially in rural areas, outreach from primary care to the community, and from secondary care to primary care and so to the community, is not systematically possible unless transport is available. This not only needs to be provided, or subsidised, but must also be appropriate to the terrain and linked to maintenance contracts.

Implications for human resource development, basic training and continuing education

Sustainability

The Ministry of Health may recognise the need for more human resource, but achievement of this generally depends on close liaison with the Ministry of Finance, the Ministry of Education and the medical and nursing schools. In a few countries (e.g. Iran) the medical schools are accountable to the Ministry of Health which can facilitate implementation of health policy with implications for medical training. In countries that have no medical education, doctors and other professionals may have to be sent abroad for training, which is costly and involves wastage if trainees do not return.

Curriculum development

It is important that the professional bodies which are responsible for oversight of the undergraduate curriculum are steered to take proper account of the importance of the common mental disorders, and the importance of ensuring that an appropriate proportion of the undergraduate curriculum is devoted to their study and to the acquisition of appropriate interviewing and therapeutic skills. Similarly the nursing curriculum needs to pay equivalent attention to mental health issues.

Vocational training for primary care doctors may or may not contain a substantial input on mental health. In the UK, around half of trainee GPs devote a sixth (six months) of their three-year postgraduate training to psychiatry, but even this tends not be aligned to their future work in primary care but rather to the role of an inpatient specialist seeing the less common disorders. The content of vocational training schemes in the UK, for example, is organised by medical schools with oversight from the relevant professional colleges (associations). These should now take proper account of the necessity for all vocational training schemes to contain a significant proportion of time on mental health in primary care.

Nurse education

In Zanzibar and the mainland of Tanzania, all nurse trainees do several weeks' mental health in their third year, and all the male trainees do 12 months' psychiatry in their fourth year (the female trainees do midwifery in their fourth year). This results in nurses throughout primary care and general secondary care who are relatively knowledgeable about mental illness.

Training a cadre of community health workers in mental health skills

Several low-income countries are finding this a useful way forward in the delivery of mental health care across the population, where primary care doctors have to cover a population of 10,000 or more (Murth & Wig, 1983). For example, in Iran and Pakistan, village health workers receive several months' training in priority subjects, including the principal mental disorders (Mubbashar, 2001; Mohit, 1998). As well as their basic training, such community health workers will have continuing educational needs and a need for continuing support, supervision and quality assurance of their work.

Continuing professional education for primary care teams

Further professional education, where it exists, may be organised by the local health services. Policy needs to address levers for encouraging primary care professionals to take up regular opportunities for continuing professional development on mental health, and for ensuring the ready availability of good-quality teaching which is appropriate for primary care. This may involve access to journals, video-teaching, role-play, lectures, workshops, etc.

Facilitating levers. Courses that currently exist tend to 'preach to the converted', i.e. around 5–10% of primary care practitioners. The challenge is to persuade all practitioners to systematically update their skills and knowledge of mental health issues on a regular basis. In some countries, small incentive per diem payments are made to all primary care staff to attend regular continuing education sessions, and uptake is then often around 100%.

Such attention to small incentive payments, the basis of contracts, and any legislative framework which may be required to support and enable appropriate mental health work in primary care is therefore helpful. This is particularly important in countries where doctors' professional roles have hitherto been more influenced by government legislation than by professional bodies which may still not be sufficiently influential (e.g. in Eastern Europe).

Implications for policy on nursing education and development

Primary care nurses have a significant role to play. Primary health care in low-income countries has always relied heavily on nurses but their role is also increasingly prominent in richer countries. For example, in the UK, practice nurses working inside the primary care team (e.g. doing cervical smears, vaccinations, dressing leg ulcers, etc.) may detect mental disorder, and there is evidence that practice nurses can play an effective role in the management of people with mental disorder (Mann et al., 1998) if given appropriate guidelines. This has implications for the continuing education of practice nurses. Similarly, district nurses look after large numbers of older people who have high rates of depression, and health visitors look after young mothers who also have high rates of depression. Practice nurses also have many opportunities to promote mental health, which should be included in general health promotion. Simple self-help techniques for managing emotional distress – e.g. physical activity, talking over problems, assertiveness and relaxation – are just as important as advice on smoking cessation or diet and also have a positive impact on physical health. It is therefore important that mental health policy pays appropriate attention to the continuing professional development of primary care nurses (e.g. Abiodun, 1991; Jenkins, 1998a).

In low-income countries, it is important to give mental health education to midwives and traditional birth attendants who have the opportunity to detect and refer post-natal psychosis and severe depression. In low-income countries, where there are few medical practitioners in primary care, nurses are likely to be given responsibility for prescribing medicine, and it is important that their basic training and continuing education programme support them in this role.

Implications for supply of essential medicine

It is possible, using basic epidemiological data, to calculate the requirements for essential medicines (WHO, 1998) for a population of, say, 10,000 people, served by a primary health care unit.

Implications for policy on social care

Mental disorders in primary care carry a high disability and impaired social role performance, which means that primary care should interface well with social care, both statutory and voluntary. Primary care has the potential to provide a referral and support service to increase awareness of and access to existing sources of support within the community. This could include facilitating self-help groups, providing access to user and patient support via the internet and building links with religious organisations. Strengthening social support reduces the burden on primary care not only by mediating symptoms, but by reducing the risk of mental health problems developing. In the UK in the 1970s there were various experimental schemes to attach social workers to primary care, which demonstrated good social outcomes (e.g. Corney, 1992). No country currently has good integration of primary health and social care, but there is no doubt about the need for close interfacing (Goldberg & Huxley, 1992).

Implications for policy on education

Mental disorders are common in children, and many predispose to mental disorders in later life. Primary care is uniquely positioned to recognise and address problems in children and to support schools to play their roles, both by liaison and consultation with teachers and by contributing to the curriculum. Mental health promotion should be as integral to education as is physical health education. Schools will need policies on bullying, truancy, supporting teachers, etc. A recent study in Norway (Olweus, 1993) showed that being a bully or a victim of bullying at school is a predictor for later problems, including conduct disorders, crime and alcohol abuse (bullies) and depression, anxiety and suicidal behaviour (victims). There is therefore a strong case for including anti-bullying strategies as a key mental health promotion intervention. In some countries, e.g. India and Pakistan, school children play a vital role in recognising illness such as epilepsy and schizophrenia in adults and bringing them to medical attention (Saeed et al., 1999). In other countries, for example Zanzibar, primary care teams include health education workers who link with schools on a local basis (Jenkins, Mussa & Saidi, 1998).

Implications for policy on employment

Mental disorders are common in employed adults (e.g. Jenkins, 1985a) and primary care teams often provide the occupational health care for businesses and industries. It is vital that such occupational health care is able to address mental health problems and to work with employers to establish sensible workplace health policies, which address mental health (Corney & Jenkins, 1992; Jenkins & Warman, 1993; Department of Health, 1996a). Employers need a greater awareness of the benefits of adopting policies to promote mental health at work. A number of stress-related disorders, as well as anxiety and depression, have been linked to a poor-quality working environment. Lack of control at work also increases the risk of cardiovascular disease (Marmot et al., 1991).

WHAT FURTHER RESEARCH DIRECTIONS ARE NECESSARY FOR MENTAL HEALTH IN PRIMARY CARE?

There is a pressing need for evaluative cost-effectiveness studies (e.g. Chisholm et al., 2000) on the use of good practice guidelines in general practice to reduce the public health burden of the common mental disorders in a variety of relatively rich and low-income countries, and in the specific use of antidepressants in resource-poor countries. There is also a need to evaluate different systems of primary care in relation to the way in which they tackle mental health problems. In particular, the routine use of primary care nurses, which has been evaluated in the UK, needs to be evaluated in other countries. Hitherto, research has focused on mental illness in primary care (Ustun & Sartorius, 1995) but it is crucial that the evaluation of strategies for mental health promotion and primary prevention in primary care, for all age groups, should not be neglected (Jenkins & Ustun, 1997).

How to implement successful research findings on mental health in primary care

Implementation of successful research findings will be influenced by a number of levers for change:

- Firstly, by leadership from cutting edge practitioners who spontaneously read the journals and attend courses.

- Secondly, by advice to commission evidence-based medicine, which will be influenced by the evidence-based medicine movement and the desire of commissioners to allow it to affect their commissioning decisions.
- Thirdly, user demands as advances are disseminated into the media. The lead-in time for new treatments such as drugs, etc., is quicker than the lead-in time for new deployment of manpower because of the need to produce and skill up the relevant professionals.
- Fourthly, by incorporation of findings into routine training programmes.
- Fifthly, by use of good practice guidelines (e.g. WHO, 1996a; WHO Collaborating Centre, 2000).

CHAPTER EIGHT

Specialist care and its links with primary care

Key Points

- *Specialist care and primary care must be intimately linked.*
- *The models required will depend on the wealth and nature of individual countries.*
- *There are seven irreducible elements of care which all countries will need to deliver.*
- *There are ten components to a comprehensive mental health care system but only rich countries will be able to afford the full spectrum of specialist services.*
- *Specialist support to primary care is a useful model to ensure efficient use of relatively rare skills.*

Unless specialist mental health services are comprehensive in terms of supplying the various separate functions which are required by service users, it is likely that the missing element of the service will damage the whole service delivery strategy. For example, to supply good health and social care in the absence of housing or income for food will mean that poverty and homelessness will soon remove the benefits of health interventions. Yet the reverse scenario is equally ineffective, as without symptom control and social support, severely ill individuals may not retain housing opportunities or manage their personal finances. The importance of viewing care in a holistic way, not limited to health care needs alone, cannot be overstated (Jenkins et al., 2000).

Achieving comprehensive specialist mental health services is often conceived of in terms of delivering a large spectrum of Western-style services, with many different components of in-patient care, supported housing, rehabilitation, etc. (Strathdee & Thornicroft, 1996). While this model represents a legitimate aspiration in richer countries, where it is at least partially supported by evidence on outcomes, it will not be realistic for many low-income countries, particularly those with large rural areas.

On the contrary, attempts to invest in one part of such a spectrum may utilise all the available resources, and actually reduce overall efficiency. Even most Western countries do not have a full 'spectrum of care' in every locality. Australia, parts of the USA, and the northern European social democracies come nearest, but many of these have gaps in housing, income support and social care, for example. They still suffer from scandals concerning poor care.

Some countries have Western-style specialist services in the city and only primary care in large tracts of rural areas. Equity is therefore an important challenge.

A more widely applicable approach is to use a 'systems approach' to planning care, starting with the irreducible functions that are required, and building gradually towards more comprehensive care. In doing so, it is important to consider how these functions can be met within existing social institutions and resources. It is also often better to consider how to assist mentally ill people to access generic resources within society as a whole rather than create or build special separate facilities for them.

WHAT ARE THE IRREDUCIBLE ELEMENTS OF CARE?

There are seven irreducible elements that all care systems for severely mentally ill people will need to have or to access.

Accommodation/shelter

All mentally ill people must have some accommodation or shelter of a type considered as acceptable within the relevant society. In many cultures, families will provide accommodation, and there is no perceived need for additional support. However, even in such countries, there are often deprived subgroups, e.g. migrant workers and refugees, who have no family to take care of them, so their needs for accommodation should be considered. Even in countries where family responsibilities are taken seriously, the stigma surrounding mental illness may be so great that people with mental illness are not accepted back home after an in-patient stay. Unless accommodation is available, therefore, the patient either stays in hospital or becomes homeless.

Where family support is not able to provide housing, accommodation and shelter should usually be delivered through the normal housing mechanisms such as private or group ownership or public housing agencies. Where public housing agencies exist, they must be included in the overall strategy and must give a level of priority to mentally ill people. Where mentally ill people remain within private or group accommodation in their local community, the community itself may require support and information. Special needs housing or permanent asylum will be required for a few individuals with extremely severe needs, but cost considerations mean that it is best to minimise this requirement as far as possible.

An adequate level of income

The adequacy of income is clearly relative to the wealth of a particular country or community. However, within this context mentally ill people should have the opportunity to earn a reasonable income if they are able to work or, if they are not, to receive some income support via social welfare schemes. In countries without formal social welfare structures, attention needs to be paid to targeting a proportion of what aid and support is available to mentally ill people. The staff administering social welfare programmes need basic training and information about mental health problems. In some cases arrangements must also be made to provide support to enable people suffering from mental health problems to manage their finances by mechanisms such as setting up bank accounts for them, arranging for regular payments to be made from a reserve, or supporting them in making suitable arrangements for themselves.

Occupational and other meaningful activities during the day

Most commonly, this will be understood either as paid employment, or the ability to participate fully in community and family activities. Other roles, which can be valued, include undertaking voluntary work, study or religious duties. Valued activities will vary from society to society, but mentally ill people need to be able to take part in these activities and be supported to do so. This can be achieved through a combination of policies to fight discrimination and ensure access to employment, and action and support to help mentally ill people return to work, or to pick up valued activities after a breakdown. Such occupational rehabilitation will need to pay attention to specific work skills, interpersonal and social skills, and patients are more likely to sustain such activities if they are supported to strengthen their social networks at work and at home.

Social support

This can come from a variety of sources including informal carers and local communities. Most severely mentally ill people will, however, bene-fit from some specialist social support to enable them to participate as fully as possible and to pick their way through the legal and bureaucratic systems of the society in which they live. Support might be needed for a range of activities including accessing generic services and opportunities or help with daily living. Social support may often need to be extended to carers.

Physical and mental health care

Access to health care is needed not only in terms of primary and secondary mental health care, but also to maintain good physical health, as the physical health of severely mentally ill people is often poor. A range of treatments should ideally be available for mental health care, including medication, psychological interventions and rehabilitation programmes. Mental health care must include provision for coping with crises.

Information and communication

This is the least tangible of the seven key elements of care, but mentally ill people and their carers and families need to be told what services and support are available and to be given information about mental health problems and treatments. Carers and families must be involved in planning care.

Assessment and triage

This final element relates more to how care is organised than to its components. All care systems should provide the opportunity for patients or users to have at least a basic assessment of their needs, in which they and their carers participate, and which is used to plan their care. Given that all systems are likely to lack optimal resources, decisions will then have to be made on how to allocate scarce resources. Transparent criteria should be formulated so that this can be done fairly, on the basis of the urgency and extent of an individual's need.

WHAT IS THE BASKET OF SERVICES FOR COMPREHENSIVE CARE?

All countries will need to address the seven basic elements of care in some form, and not all countries can afford or will wish to aspire to a Western model of psychiatry. A better initial approach will be to examine how existing services and social structures can deliver the seven essential elements described above. However, it is useful for planning purposes to describe the core elements of the comprehensive care that has been developed in many countries. Strathdee & Thornicroft (1996) have developed a useful description of the main attributes of a comprehensive mental health service and have identified the ten core components listed in Box 8.1.

In their book, Strathdee & Thornicroft describe how to develop these components of services. In many countries, the more detailed basket of services to deliver these functions can be described as shown in Box 8.2.

BOX 8.1
Components of a comprehensive mental health service system
(adapted from Strathdee & Thornicroft, 1996)

1. Identification of mentally ill people and population/community needs
    assessment.
2. Care planning system.
3. Hospital and community beds/accommodation, with bed management.
4. Case management and assertive outreach (i.e. planned and sustained
    contact with individuals by community based care teams).
5. Day care, rehabilitation, education and work opportunities.
6. Crisis services.
7. Individual needs assessment and consultation/communication.
8. Carer and community education and support.
9. Support, training and development for primary care and good liaison
    between primary and secondary (i.e. specialist) care.
10. User advocacy and community alliances.

Box 8.2
The detailed elements of a comprehensive specialist mental health service

Basic element of care	Specific services
Housing/Accommodation	Ordinary housing with visits from trained support workers
	Sheltered housing where the support worker is on site
	Group homes/shared housing
	Hostels with various levels of support
	Residential homes
	High support accommodation (i.e. with trained staff available all day)
	24 hour nursed accommodation
	Acute hospital care
	Secure units with various levels of security for mentally disordered offenders
Income	Welfare benefits/aid
	Welfare advice and help in obtaining benefits
Daytime activity	Ordinary employment opportunities
	Supported employment where a trained worker provides support
	Adult education programmes
	Employment rehabilitation places
	Clubhouse (i.e. groups undertaking leisure and employment activity)
	Day centres and hospitals
	Drop-in centres
Social support	Support with daily living
	Social work or social welfare support
	Occupational therapy

Health care	Physical health care provided through the primary care system
	Crisis intervention
	Alternatives to hospital (e.g. Home treatment services)
	Assertive outreach
	Community mental health services
	Psychiatric medicine and nursing offering a range of treatments
	Tertiary services for rarer disorders
Information and communication	Written information in the user's first language
	Verbal information
	Regular contact with user and carers
Assessment and triage	Individual needs assessment
	Care planning
	Clear criteria for access
Human resources	To deliver the above

Adapted from Sainsbury Centre for Mental Health (see SCMH, 1998)

CAPACITY FOR MENTAL HEALTH SERVICE DEVELOPMENT

Specialist capacity

One psychiatrist per million population is a common scenario in low-income countries, some countries operating at one psychiatrist per 5 million or even no psychiatrist at all, compared to one psychiatrist per 50,000 population in the UK and one per 20,000 in Eastern Europe. In many poor countries and/or countries with vast rural areas, access to a specialist is geographically impossible, and the question arises how to deliver specialist support in such situations. In low-income countries specialist services are usually in extremely short supply, and therefore it is even more important to use them to best effect. Often the distribution of specialists is not equitable, relative to the distribution of the population, with most psychiatrists concentrated in the main cities for a variety of reasons, including the availability of private practice, the availability of academic links and posts, and the availability of schools and other facilities for families. For example, in Tanzania over half the country's psychiatrists live and work in Dar-es-Salaam, leaving four or five psychiatrists to care for 29 million people. A similar situation exists in Australia and many other countries. The USA and Eastern Europe have much higher proportions of psychiatrists per head of population than other parts of the world, and it is therefore important to interpret local research evaluations in the light of the specific resources of that country.

Even in rich countries, specialist mental health staff will nonetheless be in short supply relative to the mental health needs of the population and, therefore, policy must be developed and implemented to ensure their efficient deployment. Attention needs to be given to the construction of attractive posts which offer exciting and interesting work, are suitable for people with families, but nonetheless meet the overall service needs of the country.

Capacity for local service development

There are a number of issues to consider in stimulating a country's capacity for local service development.

Existing resources and infrastructure

The way in which community mental health services are delivered is highly dependent on the existing resources and infrastructure of a country. In relatively rich countries that can afford specialist staff, community care is often delivered by community psychiatrists, community psychiatric nurses in collaboration with social workers, community psychologists, and community occupational therapists – often supplemented by voluntary organisations.

In countries that cannot afford high numbers of specialist staff but do have doctors, e.g. India, the community mental health programme is delivered by doctors – both treatment and follow-up. In Nepal, where there are hardly any doctors, health workers provide treatment and follow-up at the primary health care posts. In Iran, most treatment is provided by the health worker who can refer to the GP if necessary.

Overall in poor countries, over the past few decades, there has been relatively little growth in the numbers of specialist personnel, partly because of lack of resources, and partly because of the 'brain drain' to the richer countries. For example, although India had 500 psychiatrists in 1972 and about 3000 by 1995, there was no similar increase in trained clinical psychologists, psychiatric social workers, psychiatric nurses and rehabilitation personnel (Wig & Murthy, 1994; Pai & Kapur, 1983).

Capacity to integrate community mental health with primary care

In those developing countries which have pioneered community approaches to tackling severe mental illness, most have pursued the strategy of integrating such community approaches with primary care. The stimulus for this was the WHO collaborative multi-centre international project on strategies for extending mental health care, 1975–1981, which involved seven developing countries: Brazil, Columbia, Egypt, India, the

Philippines, Senegal and Sudan (Sartorius & Harding, 1983; Murthy & Wig, 1983).

A number of other countries in Asia, Africa and South America have subsequently experimented with this approach. For example, in Columbia, ancillary nurses have been found to be able to provide care for people with non-psychotic problems. In Tanzania, a pilot programme in two demonstration areas was launched and evaluated (Schulsinger & Jablensky, 1991).

Regular training of primary care personnel about the needs of people with severe mental illness has been organised in Bangladesh, Bhutan, India, the Maldives, Nepal, Pakistan, Egypt, Yemen, Iran, Somalia, Afghanistan, Iraq, Sudan and a number of other countries in sub-Sahara Africa (e.g. Mubbashar et al., 1986; Murthy, 1983). In India, the following facilities have been developed in various regions:

- Alternative community care facilities like hostels
- Half way homes for mentally ill people to participate in social skills training
- Vocational training and preparation for community living
- Education of family members of persons with schizophrenia about coping skills, understanding the illness, crisis support and reducing family stress and burden
- Sheltered workshops for people with mental illness and learning disabilities
- Training for non-professionals to work with the different categories of mentally ill individuals (Murthy & Burns, 1992)
- Day care centres
- Crisis intervention centres utilising community volunteers
- Community level detoxification camps
- Self-help groups for families
- The use of traditional systems like yoga and meditation (Wig & Murthy, 1994).

Developing and supporting professionals to work in the community

To support the community level activities there is a need for the role of the specialist to be different from the hospital-orientated one. The psychiatrist and psychiatric nurses (and clinical psychologists and psychiatric social workers where they exist) will have to devote a significant portion of their time to supervision rather than direct patient care. They need to be able to adapt their working practices for the community rather than the protected environment of a hospital or clinic, and they need to acquire new skills and the capacity to co-ordinate complex elements of care (Murthy, 1997).

Therefore, to a support community mental health programme, training of psychiatrists should include supervised experience in the above areas. This has been one of the important recommendations of the WHO Expert Committee on Mental Health:

> Specialised mental health workers should devote only a part of their working hours to the clinical care of the patients; the greater part of their time should be spent in training and supervision of specialised health workers who will provide basic health care in the community. This will entail significant changes in the role and training of the mental health professionals. (WHO, 1975)

Para-professionals and health workers with small amounts of training may need to be given responsibility for prescribing a limited range of drugs and, if so, there will need to be mechanisms for supervision and continuing education.

Bed availability

In almost all low-income countries, there are very limited numbers of in-patient beds available for the care of the mentally ill and few specialist personnel. For example, in the South East Asian Region (India, Pakistan, Bangladesh, Sri Lanka, Nepal and Myonmar) there was only one psychiatric bed per 30,000 population (Murthy, 1983) in contrast to 2–13 beds per 1000 population in Europe (Sartorius, 1990). Zanzibar has 1 bed per 10,000 population (Jenkins, Mussa, & Saidi, 1998).

Private practice

In many countries, the availability of specialist doctors, psychologists and nurses is even less than it appears because of the time devoted to private practice in order to supplement the basic salary. Apart from availability for direct clinical work, it is also important to consider availability for audit, planning and service development and essential research. It is therefore important for countries, when determining salary structures, to consider the opportunity costs of losing a significant proportion of a highly trained specialist's time, not just from the clinical work, important though that is, but also from the strategic planning and service development function which is also essential.

The potential and actual contribution of families

Most of the recent expansion in specialist services has occurred in relation to non-institutional components. Much of the care has occurred in the family and the community. Stigma about mental illness exists and varies from community to community but, nonetheless, in many developing countries most families prefer to care for ill family members despite the stigma and lack of support which may leave families isolated or excluded. This is important for mental health planning. Families are a vital resource in the implementation of community care and considerable attention needs to be paid to ensuring that they receive adequate support and information.

Occupational rehabilitation

In richer countries, occupational rehabilitation of severely ill people back to employment and their other social roles has generally been considered the preserve of the specialist services; and rehabilitation centres have been set up in association with the specialist services. Some excellent examples are also to be found in low-income countries (Kilonzo, 1992). However, if occupational rehabilitation is to be available for most severely ill people who need it, it will have to be made available at the primary care level rather than exclusively at the specialist level as in many low-income countries. This is attributable to the great shortage of specialist care, and because even each primary health care unit covering a population of 10,000 people will have at least 50 people with chronic schizophrenia, 50 people with bipolar disorders and several hundred with severe depression to care for, with little or no access to distant specialist services. Therefore, part of the support that needs to be given to primary care is expertise in stimulating, for example, the development of local NGOs to carry out such a task in conjunction with the health care system.

Evaluation of a model programme

A useful model public mental health programme was evaluated in Guinea-Bissau (Joop de Jong, 1996). Following independence in 1974, Guinea-Bissau transformed its centralised, curative and hospital-based approach into a decentralised and preventive approach, and set up a nationwide primary health care system. The model programme had three main aspects: a small-scale psychiatric hospital for referral, training and support of the basic mental health programme; participant observation with traditional healers to explore possibilities for collaboration; and a public health approach, which was delivered in three stages:

- firstly, an epidemiological investigation to discover (a) the percentage of adults and children visiting basic health care facilities in a rural and an urban area who had a mental disorder, (b) the kind of disorder, (c) whether these problems were recognised by health workers, and (d) a qualitative and quantitative assessment of the community strengths and impediments to setting up a nationwide intervention programme;

- secondly, a training programme for health workers and repetitive supervisory visits to the primary care facilities;
- thirdly, an evaluation of the programme.

The Guinea-Bissau approach was inspired by the WHO Collaborative Study on strategies for extending mental health with primary health care (Sartorius and Harding, 1983), and according to WHO, Guinea-Bissau was the first low-income country to succeed in integrating such a socio-psychiatric programme into its basic health care services on a national level.

Using the information gathered in the first stage on prevalence, evidence of community concern, seriousness, susceptibility to treatment, sustainability of the programme, and knowledge and skills of the health workers, it was decided to construct a training programme for health staff working at the level of primary care, about psychosis, agitation, neurotic and especially depressive disorders, and epilepsy. The training programme also included the nurses who train and supervise the volunteer village health workers. The intervention also included increasing the supply of essential psychotropic medicines to the health centres.

The evaluation in the third stage showed that there was no need for a separate cadre in a basic mental health programme. Primary care nurses were successful in diagnosing and treating severe mental disorder, major depression and epilepsy. However, there was less success with somatising patients (i.e. those showing symptoms of physical illness as a result of mental health problems). The costs of the basic mental health programme are low, given that the functioning primary health care system already exists and that buildings and salaries are already funded.

The author concluded that the programme only works with supervision; the health workers only started to practise their acquired knowledge after the supervising team had visited them.

Experience elsewhere also argues that successful integration of mental health care into the general health care services in developing countries also necessitates both short- and long-term training programmes for the primary health care workers (Abiodun, 1990).

PROBLEMS IN IMPLEMENTATION

A number of countries have model projects which have not been disseminated across the whole country and it is important to explore the reasons why this might be the case. Lack of resources is obviously an important factor, but it has been argued that reasons for slow development may include:

1. Cultural resistance to either the specific explanations for illness or the implications of modernisation in general (Gallagher, 1993).
2. The absence of indigenous capital with which to modernise the existing social and economic infrastructure and to create the organisational resources necessary to establish an enterprise as sizeable as a health care system (Reich, 1993).
3. The fact that neither international donors nor local governments have hitherto considered health services to be a priority for external donor funding compared with development of the physical infrastructure or the creation of viable economic organisations (Hecht, 1995).
4. The perceived importance of physical health as opposed to mental health as a priority in developing societies serves to restrain the growth of mental health systems (Desjarlais et al., 1995; Harpham, 1994).
5. Countries may like to retain examples of modern services for their symbolic value as indicators of modernisation, but not to put in sufficient resources to disseminate the modern service across the whole country. Thus the new mental health service serves a symbolic rather than a functional purpose giving the country cognitive, socio-economic and political legitimacy, helping to draw resources into the country from external sources. Thus the authors argue that such demonstration sites of modern health systems will not disappear but neither will they expand to the level required to address actual levels of psychological disorder in the population (Tausig & Subedi, 1997).

Clearly then, major shifts in attitudes are required within governments, if mental health services are to achieve sufficient priority to be established systematically across a country. It is also true in richer countries that senior officials often like to say that mental health is a priority, without following it up with actual hard resource allocation of the size that is needed to meet national needs.

The Tanzania WHO intervention is an example of an evaluated pilot which was not subsequently established systematically across the country. It was a pilot implementation phase of a national mental health programme carried out as a co-operative venture between the Government of Tanzania, DANIDA and WHO in the 1980s. Although Tanzania had already achieved wide coverage of its population through a decentralised and easily accessible system of primary health care facilities providing the most essential services, its mental health services were poorly staffed and concentrated in a few custodial-type institutions and out-patient departments that were hardly capable of ensuring one contact per year to about one-fifth of the estimated 100,000 severely mentally ill adults and 37,000 children in need of care at any given point in time.

The programme design aimed to take full advantage of Tanzania's existing primary care infrastructure by integrating mental health into the general health services of the country, including the 'grassroots' level in the villages and districts.

The essential features of the strategy were to integrate mental health care within the general functions of the health workers at village and dispensary level, with the capacity to refer to specialist mental health services at district and regional levels. Four target conditions were designated as programme priorities: acute psychosis, epilepsy, common emotional illness (such as depression, anxiety, somatisation), and mental retardation.

The strategy was pilot tested in two regions – Morongoro and Moshi. For a period of three years, a WHO consultant was posted in each of the two pilot areas, and a third WHO consultant was based at the Mental Health Resource Centre at Muhimbili (Schulsinger & Jablensky, 1991).

It was intended that following the withdrawal of WHO consultants and the reduction of external financial support, the government would extend the programme to other regions of the country. This did not happen in the succeeding years, at least partly because of the government's subsequent financial difficulties. However, there are now plans to further develop mental health in primary care in Tanzania.

SPECIALIST CARE AND ITS LINKS WITH PRIMARY CARE

The availability of trained psychiatrists ranges from 1 per 20,000–50,000 in Western countries to 1 per million in low-income countries, to even 1 per 5 or 6 million in some of the poorest areas of the world. These figures, using psychiatrists as an example, demonstrate not only the wide variability in the availability of specialist services, but also that they are relatively in short supply in all countries compared to the overall prevalence of mental disorder. The challenge is therefore how best to deploy such scarce and expensive resources.

To ensure the most effective use of specialist resources and to guarantee that those in greatest need are not neglected, attention needs to be paid to the appropriate targeting of specialist resources at the more severe and difficult to treat disorders (Kingdon & Jenkins, 1996).

This requires developing agreed criteria for referral to the specialist services, taking into account diagnosis, severity of symptoms, duration and risk of harm to self or others – and also evolving safe methods of shared care, including medication, physical health care and health promotion (Strathdee & Jenkins, 1996; Lloyd & Jenkins, 1995). It is relevant to mention here some innovative strategies that there is reason to think might work. Computerised self-therapy programmes, for example, are very intriguing and have the potential to be an enormous boon in extending the number of people a single practitioner can 'treat'. The adjunctive use of self-help groups is another potentially useful strategy in which the amount of time the professional spends with each patient alone is reduced and the group is given the resources (educational tools, etc.) to take over some of the educational and support and possibly even therapeutic functions that would otherwise be met by the professional. These kinds of initiative are important if we are going to come close to having enough resources to meet the massive need for services that exists in the population (Stark, 1998; Barnes & Shardlow, 1997).

In relatively well-resourced countries, if specialist services are to be able to focus on people with severe disorders, primary care will have to look after the less severe cases. In low-income countries, primary care will need to tackle most if not all cases of mental illness. Primary care will therefore need as much back-up support from the specialist services as possible on a regular sustainable basis (Heaver, 1995) – e.g. opportunities to agree on clinical guidelines, discuss cases and opportunities to learn additional psychological skills such as behaviour therapy techniques. This is a special challenge in the many parts of the world where the population in need of treatment lives predominantly in rural areas. Problems of distance and communication and lack of availability of specialists in rural areas conspire here to create very serious problems, especially for patients with serious illness. Moving them to distant cities can result in dislocation from family and friends, and more prolonged in-patient stays. In some countries where resources are meagre, and relatives traditionally supplement the hospital diet, admission to an in-patient unit more than one or two hours' travel away may mean that a patient who stays in hospital more than a few weeks may suffer malnutrition and vitamin deficiency. Innovative models, instead of distant in-patient care, need to be developed here. New developments made possible by breakthroughs in communications technology, such as telepsychiatry and internet consultation networks, need to be considered as resources allow. However, what is most crucial is that the primary care workers should feel supported by the specialists and should feel they have adequate specialist back-up. Failure to communicate effectively is often aggravated by stigma and leads to poor patient care and misunderstanding about the respective roles of primary and secondary care teams.

Primary health care teams need to have a certain amount of basic information about local mental health services, including an organisational chart of the local services with the names of key clinical and management staff, and maps of geographic or other boundaries; an information booklet of therapies available together with named contacts to advise on appropriate referrals is also required. Secondary care teams need specific information in the referral letters including background family and social history, details of the presenting problem, interventions tried so far with outcomes, the reason for the present referral, the specific role that is being requested of the specialist team, and the anticipated continuing role of the primary care team. Likewise, primary care teams need specific information in the reply from the specialist which should include:

- a clear management plan with objectives and expected outcomes;
- an indication of the risk of suicide;
- what the patient has been told about his or her condition, the prognosis and likely continuing disabilities and influence of the patient's life style;
- the role the primary care team is expected to play in the management plan;
- the role the specialist staff will play and who will be responsible for doing what and within what time-scale, including prescribing and monitoring roles and responsibilities.

POTENTIAL MECHANISMS FOR PRIMARY–SECONDARY CARE INTEGRATION

Specialist attachments to primary care

Numerous developments have arisen from this need, and some have been evaluated in a number of countries. They have generally built on the practice of attaching specialist personnel to the primary health care (PHC) team.

Social workers

For example, schemes of attached social workers have proved to be of value in the treatment of people with chronic depression related to social difficulties (Corney & Jenkins, 1992). General social work in primary care in the USA has been reviewed by Henk (1989). However, a recent study by Badger et al. (1997) suggests that the majority of rural primary care physicians in the USA have not considered hiring a social worker for their practice.

Community psychiatric nurses

Community psychiatric nurses (CPNs) were developed in the 1970s to support people with severe mental illness. Community psychiatric nurse attachment to primary care teams became a common scenario in the UK, despite little evaluation until Gournay & Brooking (1995) demonstrated the enormous opportunity cost entailed in thereby withdrawing CPNs from the care of severely mentally ill people. The 1990 quinquennial review of CPNs in England showed that three-quarters of CPNs had no one with schizophrenia on their books and three-quarters of people with schizophrenia were not in touch with a CPN. Following the ministerial mental health nursing review which called for a greater targeting of CPNs on people with severe mental illness, the 1994 quinquennial review of CPNs showed that where CPNs received referrals from psychiatrists, 80% of their case load was made up of people with severe mental illness, almost the converse being true in those who took their referrals from GPs.

Psychologists

Schemes of attached psychologists have been evaluated in the treatment of anxiety disorders, and in cognitive therapy of depression (Robson et al., 1984). Pollin & DeLeon (1996), Shapiro & Talbot (1992) and Nicholson (1995) have recently set out psychology's potential role in integrated health delivery systems.

Psychiatrists

Strathdee & Williams (1984) found that almost 20% of psychiatrists and their junior staff were spending at least one session per week in primary health care (PHC). Three models of attachment were common. The consultation models occurred where the specialist went to the surgery and the PHC team presented patient histories of 'difficult cases'. The shifted out-patient clinic described the models whereby specialist clinics shifted from the hospital to the GP's surgery. However, the mode of implementation of these clinics was vital to their success. Where specialists and GPs met regularly, the opportunity to discuss cases at close proximity resulted in mutual learning. In well-established clinics the whole PHC team became involved in working with the specialist to provide improved services. These outreach clinics had developed in a number of models.

What should these specialist-linked attachments do?

Logistical constraints to equity

The wholesale shift of specialist personnel into primary care to do hands-on work poses a variety of risks which can be seen by the examination of the logistics of the situation. For example, in the UK there are approximately 30,000 GPs, each with an average list size of 2,000, who will on a conservative estimate have around some 300–600 people with depression and anxiety at any one time and about seven people with chronic psychosis. There are about 2,000 consultant psychiatrists. Therefore, each psychiatrist needs to have close links with at least 15 GPs (in fact, more usually 25, when one takes into account sub-specialisation) otherwise the system is not equitable. All too often you find one or two fortunate GPs receiving an intensive service, and the remainder receiving very little. If the attention of the psychiatrist is spread equitably, then it is clear that each psychiatrist can only help each GP in a hands-on way with a small number of his or her depressed patients.

A balance of activities

Thus it is clear that any proper analysis of the value of these attachments needs to look not only at the individual patient outcomes for those patients seen by the attached specialist, but also at the opportunity costs of the attached specialist's time being used in that particular way. By and large it makes more sense for the attached specialist to divide his or her time between a number of activities, including hands-on work with very difficult patients, shared care and consultation activities, and direct teaching of special skills, i.e. a supportive and educational role rather than a direct hands-on role in relation to people with common mental disorders.

Integration should not mean diversion from those in greatest need

Integration should not mean diverting scarce highly trained specialist resources from the care of those in greatest need. Rather it should focus on an appropriate relationship, which allows primary and specialist care to be each deployed to best effect to achieve maximum benefit for the population. It is therefore essential to strengthen the basic and continuing training of the various members of the primary health care unit by knowledge of assessment, diagnosis, management and criteria for referral of people with mental disorders to secondary care. This is as essential in the developed world as it is in low-income countries.

Integration via training of primary health care workers

The most effective way mental health care can reach the high proportion of people living in distant rural villages is by providing mental health training in the PHC setting, as is being done in India, Pakistan, Iran and elsewhere.

Integration via guidelines

Primary care and secondary care are more efficient and effective if there is good communication between them, agreed criteria for referral and discharge, agreed guidelines and mutual support. This is likely to entail regular meetings between primary health care teams and specialist staff to discuss criteria for referral, discharge letters, shared care procedures, need for medicines, information transfer and any other co-ordination issues, train-ing, good practice guidelines and consideration of appropriate research.

Good practice guidelines are helpful educational tools for ensuring that best practice is routine. They may cover assessment, diagnosis, manage-ment and criteria for referral. A number are available, for example the WHO ICD-10 primary care guidelines (WHO, 1996) and the UK GP Toolkit (Armstrong, 1997), but all will need to be carefully adapted for the local situation (e.g. WHO Collaborating Centre, 2000), particularly in relation to the availability of specific treatments and medicines, and in relation to the availability of specialists for onward referral (WHO, 1996; Armstrong, 1997).

Integration via management framework

Via communication. Primary care and secondary care are more efficient and effective if there is good communication between them, agreed criteria for referral and discharge, agreed guidelines and mutual support. This is likely to entail regular meetings between primary health care teams and specialist staff to discuss criteria for referral, discharge letters, shared care procedures, need for medicines, information transfer and any other co-ordination issues, training, good practice guidelines and consideration of appropriate research. Communication between primary and secondary care is an important aspect of the continuity of care. Bindman et al. (1997) investigated patients' and general practitioners' views on integration between primary and secondary services in the care of severely mentally ill people, and found considerable discontinuities of care between primary and secondary care in 100 patients in inner London.

Via provision of essential medicines. If primary care teams are effectively to look after the majority of people with mental disorders they need an adequate supply of essential medicines. This is not normally a problematic issue for developed countries but in low-income countries it is common to find that primary care units, each looking after a population of roughly 10,000 people – including 50 people with chronic schizophrenia, 50 people with epilepsy and several hundred people with severe depression – may have access to little or no medicines for their patients. They also need access to occupational rehabilitation services and to psycho-social intervention skills.

Recommendations and solutions for policy on primary–secondary care integration

At national level, policy on primary care for mental health will need to set out the goals and mechanism by which the existing primary care system will incorporate a substantial mental health component into its work in a systematic way. These mechanisms may include supporting the primary care team, firstly, by appropriate basic and continuing training; secondly, by the development and use of good practice guidelines; and, thirdly, by regular meetings with specialist staff to discuss criteria for referral and discharge letters.

A *staged service development approach* to improved working between primary and secondary care services will involve the consideration of four key questions:

- What are the needs of patients in each of the main diagnostic or client groups?
- What mental health strategy will meet those varied needs?
- How can the primary care team be optimally skilled in its own role as provider?
- What models of shared care, communication and liaison should be in place between primary health care teams and specialist services?

In order to answer these questions it is necessary for the primary and secondary care teams to come together to agree the definition of the client group to be served, to identify the needs of service users, to agree measurable outcomes to be achieved, and to aggregate up the needs of clients to inform service planning. It is then possible to plan and develop service structures appropriate to local morbidity and resource levels, to negotiate and manage the necessary changes with a feasible time-scale for implementation, and to train staff in the necessary clinically effective interventions.

Local planning of primary–secondary care integration

As a first stage in local planning of primary–secondary care integration, it is important to collect information on a number of variables, which include the number and distribution of primary health care units, centres or teams. Data on the geographical areas is relevant in calculations of likely morbidity: inner city and urban areas will have higher morbidity, while rural areas will have less. Likewise practices which are responsible for local group homes, hostels, or other mental health facilities will have increased morbidity. Information on staffing, skill-mix and levels of training of the PHC team is important and should be aggregated with data on the number, nature and training of any attached sessional staff such as counsellors, psychologists, nurse facilitators, therapists, and CPNs. Information should also be obtained on local service configuration and on the historical development of local funding and management arrangements.

Local needs assessment

Both primary and secondary care teams will need an analysis of local morbidity patterns by prevalence, severity, disability and degree of risk. They will need to have good information on the existing numbers of referrals to specialist care, the numbers and characteristics of hospital admissions, the patterns of psychotropic prescribing and costs. It is helpful to know whether there are existing practice policies for the mentally ill or prescribing or management protocols. They need an assessment of the current level of information technology in primary care units and the specialist services, and whether there are existing case registers for severe illness. Finally, they will need to analyse the existing skills and the continuing training requirements of the primary and secondary care staff.

It is only by undertaking this level of analysis that a true understanding of the resources needed to support each individual primary care team can be identified. For example, practices in an urban area or near to a large mental hospital will have larger numbers of people with severe mental illness. Practices no further apart than 100 yards can vary ten-fold in their prevalence of severe mental illness, if one is responsible for the local accommodation for people with severe and chronic mental illness who require high levels of nursing support on a daily basis.

Integration with social care

In the UK, traditionally, the majority of community mental health teams serve sector populations of around 45,000 to 50,000 people, and around 25 GPs grouped into five to ten practice teams, with boundaries co-terminous with local authorities. Increasingly, best practice is seen as integrated health and social care teams, with sessional input from welfare benefits advisers and special needs housing workers working to serve a grouping of primary care practices. The development of Primary Care Groups in the UK (these are large groups of individual practices which collaborate for the purpose of commissioning health care on behalf of their locality) means that the likely population size for planning purposes is 100,000 to 200,000. This will have a significant impact in terms of economies of scale for specialist services.

Integration with case management and assertive outreach

To achieve optimal clinical and social outcomes and efficient service use for people with severe mental illness it is essential that a case management and assertive outreach function is available. In deprived inner city areas where there is often a high proportion of people with severe mental illness living alone, it has been argued in Western countries that it is likely that only a specialist dedicated case management and assertive outreach team will be able to provide adequate care (Wood & Carr, 1998; Stein & Test, 1980; Hoult & Reynolds, 1988). However, many teams, are establishing joint case registers with local primary health care teams, and regular joint review of the care plans, which provide an effective method of primary–secondary care integration. Especially in well-developed countries where information and computer systems are more sophisticated, there is an opportunity to build in recall systems for those requiring depot medication and regular prescriptions. Should patients fail to attend for regular review, there is then a mechanism to identify those who need assertive outreach, perhaps by the practice nurse, GP or district nurse.

In low-income countries, where there is little or no access to specialist care, such an assertive outreach function will need to be performed by members of the primary care team. It may sometimes be useful to engage in closer dialogue with traditional healers who often see many people with severe mental illness and to set up systems of shared care. There are already well-developed systems of collaboration with traditional birth attendants and orthodox care for childbirth.

Case registers which straddle primary and secondary care

The primary care team needs to have an up-to-date register or list of all patients with a severe mental illness so that they can ensure delivery of care, including the following key activities. All referrals to secondary care should receive a proper assessment and care plan. While in many instances, only a single professional needs to be involved, in more complex cases care needs to be co-ordinated. A single individual, the key worker, should be nominated to be the key point of contact with the primary care team. The key worker needs to agree the frequency of regular physical health care reviews, given that people with severe mental illness have severe physical morbidity. If there are group homes and hostels in the area, then it is important for the primary and secondary care teams to jointly agree the protocol for clinical responsibilities. It will be helpful for each primary care team to have a named liaison specialist worker whom they can contact if they need a discussion about a resident in a group home or hostel (Kendrick et al., 1991).

Key workers

If the primary care team is working in a relatively wealthy country where each person with severe mental illness has a specialist key worker (a community mental health worker, each of whom works with a small number of primary care physicians, and looks after all their patients in the community), then it is important that the primary care team get to know the relevant key workers, and develop a mechanism for making their primary care input and perspective into the care planning and reviewing process.

Shared care plans

For a number of patients, it makes good sense to share their care between primary care and the specialist team, so that, for example, the patient attends primary care on a weekly or monthly basis for regular support, medication, assessment of side-effects and continuing symptomatology; and then attends specialist care less frequently for more detailed review, or when a crisis develops. In order to ensure that such a system is well coordinated and works well for the patient without ambiguity or role confusion, it is helpful to draw up shared care plans which detail each person's specific tasks and responsibilities. These shared care plans need to be regularly reviewed and adjusted as the patient's needs change and evolve.

Availability of medicines

However wealthy a country is, there will be some financial constraints, and it is important for the primary and secondary care teams to jointly explore the financial implications of the newer more expensive psychotropic agents as well as their health and social benefits. There is a need to consider the costs of medication against improved 'compliance' or collaboration with medication, the absence of side-effects and need for anti-cholinergic medication, likely decrease in self-medication with illicit and damaging street drugs, quality of life, rates of relapse and use of expensive hospital admissions and reduction in social disability. In many low income countries, it is still a challenge to provide the bare necessities of psycho-tropic medicines for people with severe mental illness.

Particular issues

People with chronic severe mental illness

From the point of view of good outcomes, people with severe mental illness should be cared for as close to home as compatible with health and safety of the individual and the safety of the public, and in the least restrictive environment that is possible, with due regard to their rights as a human being and respect for their dignity, religion and culture. The precise service structure and configuration needs to be determined in the context of local needs, culture and resources. Services may, if affordable, include a small flexible mixture of acute in-patient beds (with bed management strategies to keep the number of expensive medium secure and in-patient beds as small as possible), halfway houses, respite houses, out-patient clinics, occupational rehabilitation, day care, occupational therapy and social activities aimed at promoting each individual's self-determination and personal responsibility in order to achieve the highest attainable level of health and well-being. It is particularly important to emphasise rehabilitation back into the normal pattern of daily activities of the rest of the population. To achieve this, it is essential to adopt strategies to reduce the fear and misunderstanding of mental illness.

People with acute psychosis and severe neuroses

To achieve optimal clinical and social outcomes for acute psychosis and severe neurosis, it is essential to have mechanisms for rapid assessment and essential treatments, including psychotropic drugs and psychological interventions. In some countries this will be achieved by rapid referral to the specialist team, in others it will be delivered by the primary care team, supported by close liaison with the specialist team, appropriate continuing training, good practice guidelines and an adequate supply of essential drugs. Close liaison with primary care results in more referrals and, therefore, higher treated incidence and prevalence rates (Amaddeo et al., 1995).

People with common mental disorders

To achieve optimal outcomes for people with the common mental disorders of depression and anxiety, it is essential that primary care teams have access to, and training in, locally adapted and agreed good practice guidelines on assessment, diagnosis, management, criteria for referral and methods of shared care if necessary (e.g. WHO, 1996a; WHO Collaborating Centre, 2000).

Addictions and HIV

As with mental disorders, there are important advantages for the addiction services in being well integrated with primary care and the mental health services (Morris, 1995; Miller & Swift, 1997). These include the advantages of early diagnosis and treatment before serious consequences have set in, the advantages of being able to attend simultaneously to co-morbid psychological problems, and the advantage of developing the necessary core competencies in the primary care teams. The close links between psycho-social problems, risk-taking behaviour and HIV/AIDS also argues for an integrated approach to mental health, addictions and HIV in adolescents and young people (Berger & Levin, 1993) and their families (Feingold & Slammon, 1993).

Mass emergencies

Disaster victims are known to be a group at high risk for developing emotional problems, but little attention has been paid to the integration into primary care of mental health care for victims of disasters, especially for the medium- and long-term consequences of disasters. Lechat (1979), Pan-American Health Organisation (1981) and Lima et al. (1988) have argued for a systematic approach to education and training of primary care workers in disaster mental health, and for strategic health planning in this area.

Communication

In all countries the specialist team will need to develop and agree a communication strategy with primary care, and to contribute to the training of primary care teams. Primary care teams will need to make sure they have a resource directory of all statutory and non-statutory services, agreed criteria for referral, and an appropriate continuing training programme.

The specialist team will need to provide the primary care team with a resource directory of the specialist and other mental health resources available locally. In wealthy countries, the specialist teams may play a role in the employment and supervision of psychologists and counsellors working in primary care, and in the job description of CPNs attached to primary care.

THE MANAGEMENT OF CHANGE

Rubenstein et al. (1996) evaluated the process of implementation of a major mental health programme integration into primary care, and listed some of the factors for successful change.

- Strong, committed leadership
- Knowledgeable experienced staff
- Systematic strategic planning
- Powerful internal and external incentives
- Involvement of key stakeholders
- Focus on principles of continuous improvement
- Effective communication processes
- Willingness to negotiate and deal with conflict
- Continuous education of workforce
- Openness to evaluation and feedback
- Integration of patient care, education and research
- Commitment to producing measurable outcomes.

Some of the barriers to change include reimbursement issues in private systems, arbitrary limits set by insurers on the length of treatment that can be reimbursed, and the attitudes of the various health professionals involved (Levin, 1993).

Education for change

The aim of integration of mental health services into primary care has major implications for basic training of doctors whose attitudes to integration are profoundly influenced by their experiences during training (Badger & Rand, 1988). This is best exemplified in the basic training of doctors in Manchester developed by David Goldberg.

CHAPTER NINE

Inter-agency working

Key Points

- *Effective inter-agency working is fundamental to the delivery of good mental health care and mental health promotion.*
- *There are 14 core issues which must be tackled in all countries.*
- *There is no 'quick fix' to achieve good inter-agency working, it requires continuous attention whatever the national health care structures.*

In all countries, a variety of agencies will be concerned with mental health, or with providing core services, whether specialist or generic, to people with mental health problems. Some of these agencies and types of agencies are listed on page 25. They include the health, social, NGO, education and criminal justice sectors. In order to deliver mental health promotion and effective services for people with mental illness, these agencies need to work together at national, local and regional level.

This chapter sets out the 14 core issues that have to be addressed in order to make inter-agency activity function well, with examples of action which might need to be taken at the three levels of activity: national, regional and local.

The importance of inter-agency working with police and with prisons is emphasised.

THE CORE ISSUES IN INTER-AGENCY WORKING

Issue 1: Boundaries and structures

All countries will have slightly different boundaries and structures in terms of how mental health agencies are organised and how the other generic support agencies are structured. For example, some countries will have mental health agencies looking across the life span. Others will organise services and structures into age groups (e.g. services for elderly mentally ill people) or to address other specific groups (e.g. workers). Some will organise according to settings (e.g. community versus hospital) or function (health versus social care). None of these systems is inherently right or wrong. In addition, different service functions may be delivered by services with different accountabilities. Some may be delivered by the independent sector, some by public bodies with local accountability and some by government. These boundaries can create all kinds of difficulties in terms of communications, planning and delivering unitary care packages. Organising all services into unitary mental health agencies will not necessarily help, as it will create new boundaries, although some countries have found this approach helpful. All countries will, however, need to analyse current boundaries and develop strategies for cross-boundary working. Possible actions:

- *National:* Set up a pan-governmental working group on mental health.
- *Regional:* Monitor local joint working.
- *Local:* Establish joint local action plans across the relevant agencies.

Issue 2: Primary care/secondary care

A key boundary in most systems will be between *primary care*, which is regarded as the local frontline of care and the first port of call for the patient, and *secondary care*, which is in the out-patient clinic and hospital run by specialist staff. However, the situation is often more complex. In some countries, there are several layers to the primary care system, e.g. in Tanzania, there are three layers: first aid workers for around 50 families, dispensaries for up to 2,000 population, and the primary care clinics for 10,000 population. Iran has two health workers for 2,000 population and primary care clinics for 10,000 population. In some countries, the secondary care staff are no better trained in mental health than the primary care staff. This boundary between primary and secondary care is usually most obvious in health care, although other social services may also split into primary and specialist elements (e.g. housing). Wherever this split exists, action is required to ensure that staff can work across these boundaries. Possible actions:

- *National:* Promulgate good practice on managing this interface.
- *Local, Regional and National:* Establish joint training for staff, develop and disseminate protocols, define patient care pathways/referral routes and set up common information systems.

Issue 3: Planning cycles

Planning cycles are often different for the different agencies. As far as possible they need to be the same, but this cannot always be achieved. However, it is important that all key staff understand the planning cycles of other relevant agencies. Possible actions:

- *National:* Establish common planning cycles where possible. Disseminate information on planning cycles across all agencies

Issue 4: Lines of accountability

As already stated, the different agencies involved may be responsible to different bodies, including local and national politicians and electorates, shareholders, trustees, religious hierarchies and foreign aid agencies. It will probably be impossible to achieve common accountabilities across all agencies, although the all-embracing mental health authority/mental health provider agency goes a considerable way towards this. Clear policy and planning by government helps to stop the various agencies pulling in different directions. However, a centralist model will not be appropriate for all countries, and local accountability sharing represents a strong alternative model. Possible actions:

- *National:* Establish a clear government policy and service framework for mental health.
- *Regional:* Ensure that regional structures work together to monitor and, if necessary, enforce this framework.
- *Local:* Establish local mental health agencies (particularly important in countries with strongly devolved health and social policy, which do not wish to use a centralist model).

Issue 5: Markets and pseudo-markets

Many countries have established markets in health and social care, even in previously strong corporate/socialist systems. The advantages of such a model have often been overstated and there are examples of the strong pursuit of such systems fragmenting and damaging mental health services. However, such systems do have advantages in terms of clarity, monitoring and possibly incentives to quality. Where they exist it is important to ensure that commissioning is co-ordinated, particularly across health and social care, and that providers are allowed to co-operate in providing integrated care packages. It should be noted that there are dangers, however, in one provider running both hospital and community care as resources tend to be swallowed up by the hospital element of the service. Possible actions:

- *National and Regional:* Encourage co-operation with the aim of integrating care for users.
- *Local:* Establish joint commissioning and, where appropriate, provider co-operation and integrated providers.

Issue 6: Financial and information systems

Different agencies will have different basic financial and information systems. These need to converge as far as possible, recognising that this takes time. Possible actions:

- *National:* Establish a national minimum data set and minimum requirements for financial and information systems.
- *Local:* Seek local agreements on standards and compatibility.

Issue 7: Good practice protocols and integrated care models

There are examples of countries where parallel agencies operate different standard care systems or work to different guidance or protocols when dealing with the same client groups or individuals. This does not work. Staff who work together delivering care to the same individual need to work to the same care model. It is important to bear in mind that delivering integrated care to individuals is not the same as integrating services. Possible actions:

- *National and Regional:* When establishing and monitoring national good practice models, care planning systems or protocols, do so on an inter-agency basis.
- *Local:* Establish local agreements on best practice.

Issue 8: Agency size and co-terminosity

Where different agencies, which have to work together, cover different geographical areas, it can cause endless problems in joint working. Realistically, however, it is not possible to reconfigure boundaries overnight to deliver co-terminosity (i.e. relevant agencies having responsibility for the same geographic area). However, whenever restructuring or reorganisation takes place, co-terminosity should be a major deciding factor in the chosen configurations. Possible actions:

- *National:* When restructuring relevant agencies, consider the implications for co-terminosity.

Issue 9: Perverse and positive incentives

Whatever financial arrangements are set up across agencies, there are likely to be incentives, some of which will be perverse. For example, where health and social care budgets are separate, it is to one agency's advantage for the other to pay for any particular patient's care. This can lead to beds in hospitals being blocked because no one wants to fund accommodation elsewhere, even though this is cheaper. Perverse incentives can be dealt with in a variety of ways – for example, by pooling budgets to remove the possibility of cost shifting or by creating positive incentives to good practice. This latter course has been adopted in Sweden where social care agencies pay for avoidable hospital care. Possible actions:

- *National:* Analyse perverse incentives and take action to minimise them.

Issue 10: Shared and joint training

Whenever staff have different training or professional backgrounds (e.g. doctors, nurses, social workers) they tend to acquire different models of mental health and different attitudes towards care delivery. This is not bad in itself, but can sometimes create barriers to communication and the integration of care. The most important way of tackling this is to develop programmes of joint and shared training which bring staff from different backgrounds together, often to update themselves on the practicalities of care delivery. Possible actions:

- *National:* Establish national programmes of joint and shared training.
- *Local:* Organise local shared and joint training events to address key issues of local concern.

Issue 11: Lead officers/agencies

It needs to be clear, within each organisation, who is the lead officer for mental health and, locally, it needs to be clear which organisation and which individuals are responsible for taking action forward. Possible actions:

- *Regional:* Require local agencies to take on stated lead roles.
- *Local:* In local action plans, designate lead agencies and individuals.

Issue 12: Mental health authorities

As already stated, some countries have created mental health authorities or agencies, either to commission all local or regional mental health services, or to provide them (or both). This model allows clear leadership and accountability, as well as limiting communication difficulties and minimising perverse incentives. However, in many countries any attempt to move towards this model will cut across existing structures and might create organisational turmoil when the focus should be on developing better services and undertaking mental health promotion. Caution is therefore probably the appropriate response to any suggestion that radical structural change can deliver better mental health services.

Issue 13: Creating the national lead agencies

This is similar to Issue 12, but at national level. There may be a case for developing a lead agency approach both to mental health policy development (which may often be placed with the Health Ministry) and to other issues, such as professional development or quality control. There may well be benefits in creating a national quality agency for mental health or some kind of national institute of mental health, but the arguments will vary from country to country. Any such agency requires a clear focus and role and strong leadership.

Issue 14: Continuing policy co-ordination over time

This is a major challenge, as national or local agreements can falter when individual officers or the political environment changes. It is worth considering embedding a requirement to work together in law, or creating long-term procedures for co-operation. Again, clear goals are required for any procedures created if effort is not to be diverted from the underlying mission. Possible actions:

- *National:* Consider the creation of a permanent national policy forum for mental health.
- *Local:* Consider creating a statutory local forum involving the key agencies to agree local plans.

In addition it is important to consider . . .

Inter-agency working with police

Policy needs to provide a framework for health staff and police to co-operate to ensure that people with mental illness who come into contact with the police receive speedy assessment and treatment. Police may be helpful in bringing acutely disturbed patients to the attention of the health service. However it is not acceptable for people with mental illness to spend long periods in a police cell. Thus, there needs to be liaison, leadership and agreement at a senior level between the Ministry of Home Affairs responsible for the police and the Ministry of Health. This needs to provide a framework for liaison between primary care teams, out-patient clinics or outreach teams and the police. Education and the establishment of agreed procedures for the police officers is important (Department of Health, 1996b).

Inter-agency working with prisons

Where possible, offenders with severe mental illness should be treated in hospital rather than in prison. Policy needs to address the principles and mechanisms of diversion of mentally disordered offenders from the criminal justice system into the health care system and the implications of this for specialist services. Offenders with less severe mental disorders will need to receive treatment while remaining in prison. Liaison with, and education of, prison staff about depression and management of suicidal risk is essential. In this context, good practice guidelines may be useful (WHO Collaborating Centre, 2002).

CHAPTER TEN

Tackling the mortality of mental illness

Public health measures to reduce suicide and
homicide by mentally ill people and to tackle
their physical health

Key Points

- *Mental illness is often regarded as not having a significant mortality but in fact it has a very substantial mortality.*
- *Suicide is a common event and a major public health issue.*
- *Most suicides are preventable.*
- *Homicide by mentally ill people is rare but its press coverage can encourage stigma.*
- *A number of measures can be taken to reduce the risk of homicide.*
- *Physical morbidity in people with severe mental illness is high. They require physical health promotion and good access to physical health care.*

It is often assumed that mental illness does not carry a significant mortality but research has shown that this is not the case. It is certainly true that the greater part of the burden of mental illness arises from its morbidity rather than its mortality, but nonetheless the mortality of mental illness is high and much can be done to reduce it.

SUICIDE

Government health policies usually aim to protect, promote and improve health and to reduce premature avoidable mortality. Premature death from suicide is a significant cause of mortality around the globe – official suicides alone form the tenth leading cause of death in the world, equivalent in magnitude to deaths from road traffic accidents or to deaths from malaria. Furthermore, we know that in all countries there is a greater or lesser degree of stigma attached to suicide, and therefore not all suicides are recorded. Epidemiological autopsy studies in a number of countries suggest that the magnitude of unofficial suicides is also very great. Premature death from suicide has many adverse consequences; in addition to the direct loss of life there is the consequence for the family of the loss of a breadwinner and parent, the long-lasting psychological trauma of children, friends and relatives and the loss of economic productivity for the nation. It is therefore long overdue that governments should take steps to reduce the mortality from suicide.

Most people who kill themselves are psychologically disturbed at the time. There is current debate about whether this is true in such countries as China and Sri Lanka where suicide rates are very high, and are particularly high in young women (Phillips et al., 1999). It may be that actions that would be non-fatal suicide attempts in the West are fatal in the East because of the easy availability and use of pesticides, for example, and the low access to medical care. The UN has called for all countries to have a national suicide prevention programme.

The World Health Organisation has identified suicide as an increasingly important area for public health action, and has issued guidelines to Member States in order to develop and implement co-ordinated comprehensive national and international strategies. In 1989, the World Health Organisation recommended that Member States should develop national preventive programmes, where possible linked to other public health policies and establish national co-ordinating committees. Its approach was based on identification of groups at risk and restricting access to means of suicide.

The United Nations has also identified suicide as a major priority. In a report published in 1996 based on a meeting involving 14 countries, it acknowledged that suicide was a global tragedy involving at least a half million victims per year (acknowledging the problem of under-reporting), and one where the trend was upward, particularly among younger age groups. One consequence of this trend has been that in the majority of countries suicide now ranks among the top ten causes of disease for individuals of all ages and among the three leading causes of death for adolescents and young adults. In some countries, suicide is the leading cause of death for those in their late twenties, and in many countries is higher than deaths from motor vehicle accidents.

The UN report proposed that most cases of suicide were preventable and that a national focus on both the behaviour and its antecedents was called for. It noted that comprehensive national strategies existed in only a few countries and proposed that such national strategies were necessary to achieve change. It also proposed that implementation and evaluation of such strategies required the establishment of a national co-ordinating body. Importantly, it advocated the development of a conceptual framework, which allows easy identification of intervention targets. It suggested that one such framework was the traditional public health model of attention to host, environment and agent. 'Host' referred to potential suicide victims who could be readily identified, e.g. at-risk populations and suicide attempters. At the environmental level, factors such as social support, homelessness, poverty, unemployment, legal sanctions, and community attitudes including stigma, which contributes to increase vulnerability of 'host' groups, can be targeted. At the 'agent' level, the prime methods of intervention are education about suicide and restriction of the means of suicide.

A number of countries are now developing suicide strategies (Taylor et al., 1997; Jenkins & Singh, 2000c,d).

As well as the important focus on national population measures to reduce suicide, it is important to remember that a substantial proportion of suicides occur in people with severe mental illness who are being cared for by specialist psychiatric services, and there are a number of important steps which services can take to reduce this risk (Department of Health, 2001). These include:

- Regular staff training (at least every three years) in the management of suicide risk and risk of violence, and management of co-morbid substance abuse.
- All patients with severe mental illness and a history of self-harm to receive the most intense level of care within the hospital.
- Individual care plans to specify action to be taken if patient is non-compliant or fails to attend, and efforts to prevent loss of contact with vulnerable and high-risk patients.
- In-patient wards to remove all likely ligature points.
- Follow-up within seven days of discharge from hospital for everyone with severe mental illness or a history of self-harm in the previous three months. (Where specialist human resources are spread too thinly to achieve this, as will be the case in many countries, efforts should be made to support primary care to assume this role of immediate aftercare.)

Primary care is a vital element of any suicide prevention strategy, as most people who kill themselves have recently consulted primary care, so opportunities for prevention exist. It has been shown that educational programmes for primary care teams about the assessment and management of depression and suicidal risk are essential (Rutz et al., 1989, 1990, 1995).

TABLE 10.1

Measures to reduce the levels of suicide: a suicide prevention strategy

Steps in pathway to suicide	Specific actions to prevent suicide
Factors causing depression	Policy on employment, education, social welfare, housing, child abuse, children in care and leaving care, substance abuse. Media guidance, public education. School mental health promotion (coping strategies, social support, bullying). Workplace mental health promotion. Action on alcohol and drugs. Action on physical illness and disability.
Depressive illness and other illnesses with depressive thoughts	Support of high-risk groups (occupational, bereaved, unemployed, painful disabling illnesses, etc.). Professional training about prevention, prompt detection, assessment, diagnosis and treatment. Improved access to mental health services.
Suicidal ideation	Good risk management in primary care.
Suicidal plans	Taboo enhancement. Good practice guidelines on looking after suicidal people in primary and secondary care.
Gaining access to means of suicide	Controlling access to means of suicide, e.g. guns, pesticides, paracetamol, chloroquine. Reduction of disinhibiting, facilitating factors such as alcohol.
Use of means of suicide	Prompt intervention. Good assessment and follow-up of DSH and suicide attempts.
Aftermath	Audit and learn lessons for prevention. Responsible media policy. Essential research and development.

HOMICIDE

Homicide by mentally ill people is a rare event. Such homicides may represent approximately one-tenth of all homicides in a country, but this needs local assessment. Simply on the basis of the numbers involved, a major public health strategy is not justified; however, such incidents can, in many countries, have disproportionate effects in terms of raising stigma. Individual incidents themselves are of course tragic and, as with suicide, have massive consequences going beyond the victim and the perpetrator.

Some action on this issue needs therefore to be considered as an integral part of the national mental health strategy.

A review of inquiries (audits) of homicides by mentally ill people in England by Parker & McCulloch (1999) found that 12 factors were important in contributing to the homicide. In descending order of importance, these were:

1. Poor risk management by mental health and other services.
2. Poor inter-professional communication.
3. Inadequate care planning.
4. Ineffective inter-agency working.
5. Procedural failures.
6. A lack of suitable accommodation for patients.
7. Inadequate resources in mental health care.
8. Failure to tackle substance misuse.
9. Non-compliance with medication.
10. A failure to involve family and carers.
11. A failure to respond to the needs of people from minority groups effectively.
12. Gaps in mental health legislation.

While some of these points will be different in different cultural settings, there are some general principles that are likely to hold good – many of which are addressed elsewhere in this text. These may form the basis for a strategy to reduce homicides by mentally ill people:

1. Risk management must be improved through training, the provision of appropriate support and materials for professionals.
2. Communications between individuals and agencies needs to be addressed using the principles set out elsewhere in this text, but including the provision of an adequate communications infrastructure, training and the development of shared protocols.
3. Care planning needs to be systematic and to address identified risk factors.
4. Maximum investment is required in a range of accommodation, and also secure provision if this can be afforded. In all countries, active management of the system is required to ensure that individuals are in the right part of the system, depending on risks and needs.
5. Substance misuse programmes need to link with mental health, and substance misuse problems need to be addressed.
6. The most appropriate medication (including new anti-psychotics if affordable) should be available. Work needs to be done with the patient to provide information and encourage compliance.

PHYSICAL HEALTH

The premature mortality associated with mental illness has been extensively studied in the Western world and, to a lesser extent, in low-income countries. A detailed meta-analysis of 152 studies in the English language literature on the mortality of people with mental illness has shown an extremely high risk of premature death (see Table 10.2) from all causes of death combined – from all natural causes such as infectious diseases, respiratory diseases, neoplasms, cardiovascular disease, etc., and from all unnatural causes including suicide and other violent causes (Harris & Barraclough, 1998). As only one-fifth of these studies examined in the meta-analysis were carried out in low-income countries, more research is required in these regions and the overall premature mortality of people with mental illness in low-income countries may indeed be even higher.

In the Harris & Barraclough review, eight papers reported on premature mortality for psychiatric illness as a whole in all treatment settings, on a total population of over 50,000 from six countries (see Table 10.2). Combining the studies gave an overall cause of death risk 2.2 times the figure expected, and this accounted for 16% of the excess deaths. Deaths from natural causes were twice the expectation, accounting for 84% of the excess deaths. Females had a significantly higher risk than males for all causes and natural causes of death.

Table 10.3 shows the increased risk of premature death in people with different categories of mental illness, and shows that the increased risk of premature deaths is not solely due to unnatural causes, but that natural causes are also a major contributor. This is illustrated in Table 10.4 by comparing the increased risks of premature deaths from selected causes, namely suicide, infections, respiratory disease, neoplasms and circulatory disease.

TABLE 10.2
Increased risk of premature death (SMR) in people with psychiatric illness –
all treatment settings

Causes of death	SMR*	Causes of death	SMR
All causes	216	Endocrine	142
Unnatural	498	Mental	1100
Natural	203	Nervous	221
Suicide	984	Circulatory	232
Other violent	275	Respiratory	242
Infectious	203	Digestive	255
Neoplasms	120	Genitourinary	203

* The SMR is the observed divided by the expected number of deaths, multiplied by 100.

TABLE 10.3
Increased risk of premature death (SMR) in different diagnostic groups
from all causes, natural causes and unnatural causes

Diagnosis	Natural	Unnatural	All causes
Mental retardation	783	103	633
Child and adolescent psychiatry	208	313	276
Anorexia nervosa	381	1083	493
Bulimia nervosa	400	2857	938
Alcohol abuse	171	442	197
Opioid abuse	435	1261	638
Schizophrenia	137	434	157
Psychotic disorder n.o.s.	237	274	239
Major depression	106	665	136
Bipolar disorder	150	918	202
Affective disorder n.o.s.	148	798	184
Dysthymia	83	453	101
All affective disorders	134	785	171
Anxiety neurosis	83	342	96
Panic disorder	178	429	206
Conversion disorder	159	1250	197
Neurosis	153	144	151
Personality disorder	147	371	184
Attempted suicide by self	259	300	591
Attempted suicide any method	166	1914	332
Psychiatric illness in old age (without dementia)	141	103	139
Psychiatric illness in old age (with dementia)	584	32	482

People with eating disorders or substance abuse are at highest risk of early death from physical illness, closely followed by people with schizophrenia and major depression. In low-income countries the other causes of premature mortality are likely to be superseded by death from infectious diseases. For example, in Zanzibar, the likelihood of dying in the mental hospital in a year of a cholera epidemic was around 50% compared with a risk of about 25% in other years (Jenkins, Mussa, & Saidi, 1998).

Such high mortalities from infectious diseases arise partly from the vulnerability conferred by malnutrition and the poor hygiene resulting from an inadequate water supply.

These findings of the significant increased premature mortality of people with mental illness from natural causes means (a) that serious attention must be paid to physical health promotion and physical health care for people with mental illness; (b) that targeted health promotion policies should be considered, for example, healthy living with schizophrenia; and (c) that people with mental illness should be informed of specific issues such as exercise, smoking, nutrition, adequate housing in cold countries, and safe sex.

TABLE 10.4

Increased risk of premature death in people with different mental illnesses from selected causes

Diagnosis	Overall SMR	Suicide SMR	Infection SMR	Respiratory SMR	Neoplasm SMR	Circulatory SMR
Mental retardation	633	42	2021	1892	206	402
Child and adolescent psychiatry	276	306	?	?	?	?
Anorexia nervosa	493	3243	?	?	?	?
Bulimia nervosa	938	0	?	?	?	?
Alcohol abuse	197	550	114	282	145	129
Opioid abuse	638	1003	1316	1071	251	909
Schizophrenia	157	900	944	230	100	104
Psychotic disorder not otherwise specified	239	462	1103	?	110	89
Major depression	136	2124	218	153	90	95
Bipolar disorder	202	1173	40	1034	98	158
Affective disorder numbers	184	1984	1478	240	98	115
Dysthymia	101	1194	220	127	105	118
All affective disorder	171	1990	938	194	95	116
Anxiety neurosis	96	629	?	?	126	120
Panic disorder	206	750	1000	?	97	203
Conversion disorder	197	0	833	?	148	138
Neurosis	151	252	1114	228	113	129
Personality disorder	184	256	2826	?	277	28
Attempted suicide by self	591	3913	?	213	169	128
Attempted suicide by any method	332	4186	?	663	123	166
Psychiatric illness in old age (without dementia)	139	?	?	?	?	?
Psychiatric illness in old age (with dementia)	482	?	?	?	?	?
Psychiatric illness – previous in-patients, first 2 years of follow-up	314	5143	429	500	189	198

CHAPTER ELEVEN

Investing for the future

Key Points

- *National strategies are required for R&D and human resources if the overall mental health policy is to be successful.*
- *Governments will also need to provide support to service user and care groups to enable them to participate in the planning and implementation of the strategy.*
- *The existing estates and other hardware (i.e. buildings and equipment) must be taken into account in planning service development.*

RESEARCH AND DEVELOPMENT

All countries need to establish a sustainable research and development (R&D) strategy and an infrastructure to support access to research evidence produced elsewhere, in order to support its policy development and implementation programme. However, the Global Forum for Health Research (2000) has drawn attention to the fact that 10% of the world's global health research resources are directed to the health problems that constitute 90% of the world's disease burden.

There is an overall need for basic scientific research into the origins and mechanisms of mental disorder as well as for more practical research into treatments, services, implementation, effectiveness and applicability. Richer countries will wish to invest in a suitable balance and range of research to meet their needs and to contribute to scientific progress; but no country has sufficient resources for all its research needs and there is frequent debate about whether richer countries have their priorities right in the way they balance their research portfolio (e.g. National Alliance for the Mentally Ill, 2000).

Clearly, poor countries cannot meet all their own research needs. For example, biological research tends to be very expensive and may be seen as less of a priority for low-income countries which will have to rely

137

heavily on research produced elsewhere, for which they will need adequate access to libraries and the internet. However, there are some crucial questions that can only be answered by local research and should be planned accordingly. Epidemiology and mental health economics are particularly important contributors to policy and planning (Jenkins, 2001b; Jenkins & Knapp, 1996).

Overall research priorities should be defined to reflect issues of enduring importance to the local mental health programme on a 10–15-year time-scale. Funding should be devoted to research on mental health in primary care as well as specialist care.

Attention should be paid to developing researchers at the pre- and post-doctoral phases of their career, and also to developing the research capacity within the routine of the health care services and within the routine of training courses. For example, a thorough and large-scale epidemiological survey in Zanzibar was carried out by student nurses as part of their training, with minimal costs (Garssen et al., 1988).

Current research challenges include:

- The drive for increased quality in mental health care.
- The importance of co-ordination and partnership across the interfaces between health care, NGOs, social care, other governmental agencies such as police and prisons, alternative or traditional healers where appropriate, and with patients and their carers.
- Inequalities in health. There are frequent inequities in health between different socio-economic groups which need to be explored, explained and redressed.
- Effective primary care is a central requisite for a high-quality mental health service because it is in primary care that most people with mental health problems are seen. Continuity of primary care reduces hospital admissions and improves mental health outcomes. Current patterns of professional cadres, skill-mix, service organisation, basic training and continuing education, and the primary care–secondary care interface need to be studied and understood to support their capacity to respond to rapidly changing environments.
- What are the needs, objectives, targets and quality indicators for a community rehabilitation service, and what is the optimum configuration of a rehabilitation service?
- Cost-effectiveness evaluations of interventions for prevention, treatment and rehabilitation. There is a great need for cost-effectiveness studies in low-income countries (Shah & Jenkins, 2000).

In addition, there will be a number of themes that cut across other physical health priorities which countries may wish to address. For example, in relation to reducing the mortality in young men, research on prevention of deliberate self-harm and suicide, on risk-taking behaviour including alcohol-related risks, and on understanding how to involve men in decision-making about their own health are all important areas where mental health research has an important contribution. In relation to improving the overall health of mothers and infants, mental health research is particularly vital, for example on preventing post-natal depression and on supporting parents in the light of changing family and social structures.

HUMAN RESOURCES

Human resources (staff) are fundamental to mental health services which are labour intensive and largely low-tech. Most mental health systems will expend over 70% of their total resource on staffing; therefore, a national human resources (HR) strategy for mental health is an essential component of the overall mental health strategy.

The components of a national HR strategy for mental health may include:

- Analysis of present and future workforce requirements springing out of the overall strategy.
- A workforce plan, looking at the future supply of staff, overall and by professional group.
- A national training plan, covering training of new staff and continuing professional development.
- A recruitment and retention strategy to ensure that supply is adequate.
- Other mechanisms for sustaining the workforce such as health and safety at work and stress reduction.
- A strategy on pay and conditions of service.
- The development of a core competency model for key staff groups.
- The development of a national agency or function to monitor implementation of the strategy.
- The development of a set of workforce indicators and national database covering issues such as vacancies, turnover, age, gender, ethnic origin, health status, qualifications, etc.
- Liaison with professional bodies, educational institutions and other stakeholders.
- A strategy for redeployment or retraining of staff to fit any national change agenda in mental health.
- A strategy to skill up generic staff in mental health.

Different countries will face different issues in developing a sustainable HR strategy. These may include:

- Poor-quality data on the workforce, which may have to be addressed through the information infrastructure.

- Low-income countries will have difficulty in meeting all their training requirements for health and social care professionals. They will therefore need a sustainable plan for production and continuing development of primary and secondary care staff, both at home and elsewhere.
- Skills shortages may have to be tackled through imaginative strategies for recruitment and retention. The latter is particularly important in many countries as, if turnover is high, it is vital to ascertain the reasons and address them. Skill mix will have to be matched to the realistic supply of professionals – i.e. unqualified workers can deliver a lot if appropriately deployed, supervised and trained on the job, but a number of countries only have ready availability of nurses, not of other professionals. In such cases it may be possible to insert additional modules into both the basic training programme and the continuing education programme to deliver basic occupational therapy, social work and psychology skills.
- Addressing 'hygiene' factors in the workplace such as workload, stress, family friendly conditions of employment, etc.
- Ensuring a good ethnic, gender and age balance in the workforce.
- Lack of attractiveness of the field. The workforce strategy must link with mental health promotion and communications strategies.
- Ensuring that opportunities for further training and promotion are equivalent in mental health and physical health, and that staff who opt to train as mental health specialists are not disadvantaged by so doing.

GOVERNMENT STRATEGIC SUPPORT
TO SERVICE USERS AND CARERS

Box 3.3 in this book outlined some possible ways of involving service users and carers in the development of the mental health strategy. Governments may find it useful to consider the funding of self-help groups and advocacy services to develop an effective means of engagement between service users and the other stakeholders, and to ensure that service users become, and continue to be, actively involved in the planning and implementation of the mental health strategy.

ESTATES STRATEGY

After staff, the estates (land and buildings) and other hardware (e.g. IT) within mental health services represent the most significant investment of national resources. The nature of the estate can be a major constraint on the speed and exact content of service change. The importance of estate as an issue – and a possible block to change – must never be underestimated. The estate should serve the services and the patients, but too often the services and patients have to take the estate as they find it. Most countries will have a mental health service estate that falls into one of four broad categories, each of them carrying significant strategic issues when planning service development:

1. *Little existing estate.* This allows flexibility, but of course means that a move to modern mental health services may require major capital expenditure.

2. *Existing estate consists of large institutions.* This can be a major obstacle to progress as such buildings are rarely suitable for modern services either in architecture, location or organisational culture/history. However, the sites can be valuable.

3. *Existing estate consists of areas within general hospitals.* This can be a useful model for destigmatising mental health problems and making them part of the health mainstream – at least at a certain point in the evolution of services. However, it ties the fate of mental health services to that of health care generally and can result in major inflexibility.

4. *A few countries have a range of estate representing a variety of flexible resources for mental health.* They are usually rich, and even then some elements of care may be lacking. While this is a good model it will not necessarily be right for, or within, the financial reach of all countries.

In planning an estates strategy it is vital to assess the current estate from a number of points of view:

- *Location* – Is the estate near the service users/areas of morbidity, and in convenient locations?
- *Value* – How much is it worth and how much of that value can be realised for reinvestment?
- *Condition* – Is it a therapeutic environment, well designed for patients and staff alike? Is there a backlog maintenance deficit? Is it in good condition?
- *Architecture* – Is this suitable?
- *Perceptions* – Is the estate valued by patients, staff and the community?
- *Culture* – Do the main buildings embody the right culture, history and ethos for mental health care?

Having analysed the strengths and weaknesses of the current estate, it is then important to assess the key elements that must be changed or added to to deliver the overall priorities. This must be done in the light of the likely available resources, and compromise may be necessary to make progress. Possible strategies within each broad estates profile include:

1. *Little estate.* This may be a desirable state of affairs to continue in countries with little available capital where there are opportunities for

integrating or continuing to integrate service users within local communities. It should not be assumed that the right aspiration is for a Western-style mental health estate. Where hard-earned capital is available it will be important to put it into flexible resources. Ten varying and small mental health units fulfilling a number of uses may be better than a new large psychiatric in-patient facility.

2. *Old institutions.* There is a rich literature detailing the stories of the old institutions and the problems that can arise in closing them and transforming services. Closing a large institution is usually the correct option when seeking to move towards comprehensive local services, and double running of institutional care with modern in-patient and community services is very expensive. However, a plan to close an old institution can easily take 20 years to deliver. Compromise in terms of limited redevelopment on the site, for example, may sometimes prove helpful.

3. *General hospital-based care.* This model may have some advantages but services need to be linked to a range of facilities in the community. It is difficult to disinvest in hospital beds before community services are fully developed, and this can require bridging funding.

4. *Range of services.* This model is good, but the range and location of facilities requires a regular review to ensure that service needs are still being met and that the right facilities are in the right location.

CHAPTER TWELVE

Some special priorities

Key Points

- *Child and adolescent mental health services deserve particular attention. They are often underdeveloped yet such services contribute to mental health right through the lifecycle and increase the resilience of communities. Attention is also needed to maternal mental health.*
- *Mental health strategies must address the needs of carers.*
- *Specific attention is needed for the development of services for older people.*
- *Countries with a high prevalence of people with AIDS/HIV must take account of the needs of this group in the strategy.*
- *Prisons contain a high population of people with mental disorder.*
- *Mental disorder is also common in the homeless.*
- *The interrelationship of physical and psychiatric disorders means that psychiatric and general medical services need to work closely together.*
- *Substance abuse is a growing problem across the world and has a major impact on mental disorders, service use and suicide.*

CHILD AND ADOLESCENT SERVICES

Children are a nation's most precious resource yet services for children and adolescents are often the least developed and resourced. Childhood and adolescent services need to be considered in a holistic manner, incorporating: mental health promotion in schools; prevention and early detection in schools and primary care; outreach to vulnerable groups such as street children (see below); prompt management in schools and primary care; referrals to child guidance clinics for difficult cases; and, only very rarely, admission to specialist units for brief in-patient care. Child guidance clinics in many low-income countries are still relatively unusual but are becoming well established in countries such as India, supported by the academic growth of the specialty (Naik, 2001).

Particular childhood disorders that need to be considered include emotional and conduct disorders, epilepsy, mental retardation, cerebral malaria and specific learning problems such as dyslexia. It is important to develop facilities for sick post-natal mothers to be cared for with their babies, and older children with their mothers. All children with epilepsy should receive adequate medication (often in very short supply in low-income countries) and school teachers should receive training in detecting and managing dyslexia, which is a significant contributor to conduct disorder and depression in children, and to antisocial behaviour in adult life.

Schools are a key setting for mental health promotion and prevention of disorders in children, as well as for identification, treatment and follow-up of mental health problems. It may be possible for trained mental health workers to be available for some urban schools, but it is also important to train the teachers, particularly in rural areas.

Street children

In a disturbing number of countries children at a young age have lost contact with their families and are found living on the streets, nearly always in squalid, degrading and corrupting conditions. Such children are vulnerable to hunger, cold, economic exploitation, drug addiction, sexual promiscuity, sexually transmitted diseases, criminalisation, imprisonment, sexual and physical abuse, and extermination at the hands of death squads.

Health workers may be able to provide street children with food, clothing and bedding, and use the contact to begin to rehabilitate them and eventually persuade them to go into a home or hostel, or rejoin their families, and attend school and training workshops (e.g. Rane, 2000).

Orphanages and children's homes

Children's homes may contain children who have been abused or neglected, children whose home life has broken down, children with developmental delay and retardation, children with speech delay and problems in articulation, children with fits, children exhibiting severe over-activity or aggression, and children with chronic physical illnesses, physical disability and handicap. Care workers in children's homes therefore require information, support and guidance in the management of such children, and their training should include education in child development, the promotion of mental health and the management of mental health problems. Surveys of people in prisons show that they contain a significant over-representation of people who have been brought up in orphanages and children's homes, suggesting the critical importance of improving and sustaining support to such vulnerable groups (Singleton et al., 1998). In some countries in Eastern Europe, following the legacy of the former Soviet Union, many children and adolescents are institutionalised rather than given effective multidisciplinary out-patient care.

INTELLECTUAL DISABILITY

Children and adults with intellectual disability (i.e. learning disability or mental retardation) should be able, encouraged and supported to lead as normal a life as possible. Children with intellectual disability, as well as having special educational needs, often also have physical, psychological and social needs. This involves a close liaison between the Ministry of Health and the Ministry of Education. Policy-makers will need good estimates of the prevalence of intellectual handicap, and an appreciation of the possibilities for prevention of some cases – for example, in areas where iodine deficiency is a significant cause, such as in Cambodia and parts of India, where iodised salt will be preventive. Many children with intellectual disability also have specific neurological problems such as cerebral palsy and epilepsy, and essential medicines are needed to ensure that the intellectual deficit is not aggravated by these associated conditions.

The psychiatric services need to plan how they can deliver an assessment and management service not only to children with intellectual disability but also to their carers (e.g. Menon & Peshawaria, 2001). There must also be an orientation in primary health care to the needs of children and adults with an intellectual handicap and their families. This may be supported by the use of good practice guidelines on assessment and management of intellectual disability. Depending on the availability of resources, consideration needs to be given to the training of child psychologists, speech therapists and special teachers. Consideration also needs to be given to the incorporation of the problems of intellectual disability into basic and specialist training and into continuing education of primary care teams, teachers as well as specialists.

Naik (2001) describes an important pilot study in India, involving collaboration between education, health and welfare departments, where district teams – comprising a speech therapist, a physiotherapist and three special educators – were posted in each of three districts, covering 50 villages in Andhra Pradesh, to support the detailed assessment of special educational needs and to deliver a 5-day teacher training programme about meeting the educational and non-educational needs of children. The children were assessed at the end of the year and showed significant improvements in speech, social skills and scholastic performance.

Services for women

Children's cognitive and emotional development is greatly influenced by the mental health of their parents, especially the mother, and particularly when the mother is the main carer (Rutter & Quinton, 1984). In addition to the general rates of adult illness, women also experience higher rates of illness around the time of childbirth. If untreated, these disorders can severely affect the mother's relationship with her children, thus damaging the child's cognitive and emotional development. Thus, the prompt and effective treatment of post-natal depression is one of the most important preventive activities it is possible to undertake.

Mental illness can cause significant strain on a marriage, and in some cultures it is relatively easy for a person to divorce a mentally ill spouse, sometimes with difficult social and economic consequences for the spouse and children. It is therefore important that marital support and therapy should be available, which is an activity that can often be usefully delivered by an NGO.

Parenting skills have a crucial impact on the development of children, and there are programmes in a number of countries that include parenting skills in health education lessons in schools, and in health discussions with mothers and babies.

CARERS

For many people with a mental illness, family and friends provide essential care which may range from practical help such as shopping and cooking to providing emotional and/or financial support. Some carers may only be needed to assist on occasions, but others may provide a high level of care and support on a continuous basis. Carers may find their caring responsibilities difficult and stressful. For example, where carers have decided to give up their employment in order to provide care, or have missed opportunities of promotion due to their caring responsibilities, they may feel resentful, socially isolated and may also have financial worries. Such factors could affect the carer's own physical and/or mental health with the result that he or she is unable to continue to provide the same, or any, level of care. The strategy should therefore take account of the importance of carers and aim to ensure that carers are provided with adequate support.

SENSORY IMPAIRMENT

Deafness may develop before speech is learned (prelingual deafness) or afterwards. Profound early deafness interferes with speech and language development, with emotional development and with educational attainment. Prelingually deaf adults often keep together in their own social groups and communicate by sign language. For the management of emotional and conduct disorders in this group, special knowledge is required of the practical problems of deafness (Hindley, 1997).

Deafness of later onset has less severe effects, but the acute onset of profound deafness can be extremely distressing, and even a mild restriction of hearing may cause depression and considerable social disability. Deafness in older people is associated with the development of persecutory delusions.

In contrast, blindness in early life need not lead to abnormal psychological development or educational retardation in relatively rich countries, but is still likely to pose considerable difficulties and physical hazards in poor countries. In previously sighted people, the later onset of blindness causes considerable distress and depression.

Information about the emotional and developmental needs of people with sensory deficits will therefore need to be incorporated into the continuing education programmes of teachers and health workers who come into contact with children and adults with such deficits.

OLDER PEOPLE

The continuing expansion in the world's elderly population is of particular significance for mental health policies and services. As the risk of dementia increases exponentially with ageing over 65, policy-makers will need to know the age structure of the over-65 population, as well as the numbers and proportion they form of the total population, in order to estimate the prevalence of dementia in their population if local epidemiological data is not available. Depressive illness is the commonest psychiatric disorder of old age; it is twice as common as dementia in Western countries.

In Western countries, a relatively high proportion of the total elderly population is in some kind of institutional care (private, local authority or health service care). In the developing world, older people are largely supported by their families. A number of studies in richer countries have shown that the needs of the elderly who cannot fend for themselves tend not to be adequately met by the State, causing neglect (including starvation, frank abuse, hypothermia, neglect of physical illness). However, there are not as many people with dementia in low-income countries as was predicted from actuarial estimates, and there is a major concern that such people are being allowed to die prematurely. The emotional strain of caring for a demented relative is now well known and occasionally manifests in elder abuse. It is therefore important to develop services that both identify dementia and support families and professional carers.

AIDS

AIDS (acquired immune deficiency syndrome) is a severe, infectious disorder of immune functioning in which the causative agent, the human immunodeficiency virus (HIV), is transmitted by exchange of bodily fluids. It is suggested that around 50% of people with the virus will progress to AIDS within 11 years of first infection.

Transmission occurs as a result of sexual behaviour, injection of drugs with contaminated needles, or iatrogenically through exchange of blood products. The prevalence of HIV infection in people who inject themselves with illicit drugs varies widely, even between adjacent geographical areas, and depends on the extent of sharing of needles and syringes and the mobility of users. HIV enters the brain shortly after first infection and may cause malignancy, opportunistic infections, vascular lesions and encephalitis. Chronic loss of global cognitive functioning with apathy, withdrawal and deterioration of personality occurs in advanced HIV disease and is a source of great concern for patients and carers.

Psychiatric disorders in AIDS, usually adjustment reactions and persisting depression, occur with approximately the same frequency as in other major and life-threatening illness. There is a greatly increased risk of suicide. Perceived lack of social support is correlated with depression. Extensive social support is often readily available to gay men who are open about their homosexuality in Western countries, but much less to drug users. Principal diagnoses in those referred for psychiatric help are adjustment disorders, major depression, psychotic states and organic brain syndromes. Psychotic states are usually affective in nature. The treatment of depression in people with HIV is relatively straightforward, but some delusional states, particularly if complicated by AIDS, encephalopathy and drug abuse, may be resistant to antipsychotic medication. The resulting behavioural disturbance can be extremely difficult to manage in medical wards, and it is often necessary to transfer the patient to psychiatric facilities where he or she may be nursed less restrictively.

It is important that AIDS counsellors are educated and supported to help patients with psychiatric complications of AIDS, and their carers.

There is a need to plan mental health promotion in schools to reduce the risk of contracting AIDS via unprotected intercourse or drug use. There is a need to ensure that girls are supported to be assertive and confident in ensuring their sexual health and safety, but there are particular difficulties in countries where the use of condoms is not widely culturally accepted by men. As well as life skills education and mental health promotion in schools to encourage abstention from drugs, efforts are also needed to reduce harm in those who do take drugs, and to contain infection. School programmes need to be youth and media friendly, supported by figures of national status, participatory for all stakeholders (from government departments to school children), locally and community initiated and within the capacity of even the poorest school to establish. The programmes should be (a) holistic (emphasising life-enhancing activities as well as confronting life-threatening issues), (b) integrated with existing health services outside the school, (c) non-controversial (acceptable to all groups and devoid of religious, ideological or gender bias), (d) built around a core component for dealing with the major threats to children's health in general, and to their reproductive health in particular, and (e) clearly targeted with measurable outcomes. There is good evidence that school-based sex education and AIDS prevention programmes that not only emphasise the social content of attitudes, values, and the attainment of skills, but also use a participatory and active learning approach, can be successful in addressing and changing adolescent sexual behaviour (Allgier, 1993).

MENTAL HEALTH SERVICES IN PRISONS

Mental illness and suicide are much more common in prisons than in the general population (Asuni, 1986; Singleton et al., 1998; Meltzer et al., 1999; Lader et al., 2000) and, where possible, offenders with severe mental illness should be treated in hospital rather than in prison. Policy needs to address the principles and mechanisms of diversion of mentally disordered offenders from the criminal justice system into the health care system and the implications of this for specialist services. Offenders with less severe mental disorders will need to receive treatment while remaining in prison, and for this reason prison health care staff need to be familiar with assessment and management of mental disorders. Liaison with and education of prison staff about depression and management of suicidal risk is also essential. Good practice guidelines for health care staff in prison are likely to be useful, and the WHO ICD-10 primary care guidelines have recently been adapted for this setting (WHO Collaborating Centre, 2002).

THE INTERRELATIONSHIP OF PSYCHIATRIC
AND PHYSICAL DISORDERS

As well as the association of psychiatric disorders with malignancy, cardiovascular disease, respiratory disease and trauma addressed in the preceding chapter, there is also an important relationship with infectious diseases, including tropical diseases such as malaria, trypanosomiasis and leprosy, making it imperative that mental health services in tropical countries have access to general medical care and vice versa (Giel, 1978; Weiss, 1985). It is also imperative that mental hospitals are equipped with basic medicines, including antibiotics for TB and oral rehydration packs for infective diarrhoea and cholera.

SUBSTANCE MISUSE

Substance misuse causes substantial health, social and economic problems. It is prevalent in the Western world and is increasing rapidly in many low-income countries (Farrell et al., 1998; Kilonzo, 1998, Odejide et al., 1993; Saxena, 2001). Misuse is highly correlated with availability, and is associated with violence, accidents, injuries and higher rates of physical illness and suicide. Mental health strategies need to include a framework for prevention in schools, communities, workplaces and in street children, as well as treatment and rehabilitation for substance abuse (Asuni, 1990; Eliany & Rush, 1992; Berterame, 1994).

CHAPTER THIRTEEN

Traditional and religious healers

Key Points

- *Traditional healers are a major health care resource of variable efficacy world wide.*
- *People often simultaneously consult both traditional healers and Western medicine.*
- *Establishing dialogue with traditional healers is therefore important.*
- *Churches and religious groups may play an important role.*
- *Safety, efficacy and cost-effectiveness studies are a priority.*

Western medicine has had enormous success in diagnosis, medicine, surgery and pharmacology and has achieved significant advances in the field of mental health. Indeed, there was a time when many people thought that Western medicine in all its forms would eventually displace the indigenous traditional medicine in low-income countries. However, in practice, traditional healing has remained popular and is a frequently used form of health care in low-income countries for both physical and mental health problems.

There is increasing realisation both of the limitations of a purely mechanistic, symptom-orientated approach to healing and of the potential and actual significance of traditional healing. Indeed it is easy to forget that, before the advent of modern medicine, health care in Western countries was delivered by a variety of traditional healers, with variable outcomes. Most of our modern medicines are derived from plants, many of which had been known and used as herbal remedies for centuries. It is also often forgotten that traditional healing, or so-called alternative or complementary medicine, continues to be a significant force in Western countries, where homeopaths, herbalists, aromatherapists and spiritual healers are not uncommon and are sometimes consulted by people with mental health problems (Leff, 2000).

ACCESSIBILITY OF TRADITIONAL HEALERS

The traditional healing system is more accessible in low-income countries than orthodox care and will remain so for some time. In rural Tanzania, for example, the ratio of Western-trained doctors to population is 1 : 20,000 and each primary health care unit is responsible for a population of 10,000; whereas the ratio of traditional healers to population is 1 : 25 (Swantz, 1990). Thus, traditional healers play a major role in treating psychiatric disorders and constitute an important health care provider in Tanzania.

CONSULTATION PATTERNS

It has been demonstrated in a wide variety of countries that traditional and religious healers are consulted at some stage by many people with mental illness. For example, a study in Nigeria showed that patients consulting traditional healers are no different to those who consult orthodox medical practitioners either in demographic factors, presenting complaints, or proximity to services (Gureje et al., 1995). In western Kenya, more than half of the patients attending health clinics have also consulted traditional healers (Acuda, 1983). In Tanzania, studies have shown that between a quarter and a third of patients with psychiatric complaints in a primary health care setting had already consulted a traditional healer (Schulsinger & Jablensky, 1991; Kempinski, 1991; Bloch, 1991). In Pakistan, recent studies have confirmed the high prevalence of mental disorders in people consulting native faith healers (Saeed et al., 2000).

It is usually assumed that those who consult traditional healers do so prior to seeking specialist psychiatric services. However, a number also consult traditional healers for a variety of reasons, including lack of progress using Western medicine, and the desire to obtain a satisfactory explanation for symptoms (Salon & Maretzki, 1983).

It is the ease with which patients are seen to move between conceptually and ideologically incompatible systems of health care that has puzzled many observers. Janzen (1978) observed that patients often use many different types of therapy in the course of an illness. He noted that most of the significant decisions about the appropriateness of any one particular type of treatment were taken not by the patient or the healer alone, but by an ad hoc group of relatives and significant others that formed around the patient with the specific aim of 'therapy managing'. Janzen used the term 'therapy managing' to denote the process by which patients' healing processes were changed from one type to another.

During his fieldwork Janzen noted that patients were moved between healing systems on an empirical basis: if one treatment did not seem to work, another would be tried. He found that changes of treatment setting were preceded by periods of discussion within the management group, and that the varieties of treatment sought corresponded to the scope of available opinion and knowledge within the therapy managing groups of family and friends. These 'therapy managers' often hold supernatural beliefs about the origin of an illness, and do not passively hand the patient over for care. Instead, they seek treatment on an empirical, symptom reduction basis, and maintain the right to alter or add to the direction of therapy on their own terms. Thus the power balance shifts from the doctor–patient relationship, in which the doctor is dominant, to a more broadly based and democratic therapy management team.

TRAINING OF TRADITIONAL HEALERS

There is a large variety of traditional healers, some of whom undergo extensive training during an apprenticeship, while others receive very little training. Untrained charlatans are also sometimes found, particularly in rapidly growing urban areas where there is less social control. In Tanzania, for example, there is a large variety of healers and little standardisation in their recruitment and training that ranges from apprenticeship to those who believe they have the ability to heal after experiencing visions (Heggenhougen & Gilson, 1998). Traditional doctors/herbalists, who practise a herbal medicine within a spiritual context, tend to have an intensive six- or seven-year apprenticeship to acquire detailed knowledge about the herbs, their identification, indications, side effects, etc. By contrast, healers who are entirely religious in their practice, often begin their practice after a spiritual call, and have no specific training.

Advantages and disadvantages of traditional healing for mental health

The potential psychological efficacy of traditional healing has been commented on by a number of authors (e.g. Edgerton, 1980; Harding, 1975). Traditional healing is totally community orientated, and operates in the social context, with strong social support functions. Supporting social networks is known to have both preventive and therapeutic efforts.

Traditional healers may use their knowledge of community life and the cultural milieu in their practice, and they recognise the value of listening and encouraging problem-solving. Traditional healing gives weight to family consultation, family prescription, family choice of treatment, family diagnosis and family preventive measures – emphases usually lacking in modern health practice (Asuni, 1979).

On the other hand, there is little doubt that traditional healers may also harm patients under their care in a variety of ways. Examples are cited of patients who have been chained and beaten; encouraged not to take orthodox medicines that would benefit them; given herbal preparations with similar pharmacological properties to the orthodox medicines they were presently taking, resulting in overdose; and given harmful doses of herbal preparations. Furthermore, as knowledge of herbs diminishes in the village and town markets where they are sold, herbal prescriptions may be inaccurately dispensed.

ISSUES FOR COLLABORATION

Despite the difficulties arising from the variabilities in practice of traditional healers and the differing conceptual frameworks, there is increasing support for the idea of encouraging greater professional accountability and training in traditional healers and for the idea that the health services of developing countries may be sustained more effectively by integrating traditional and modern approaches to therapy. It therefore makes sense to consider and evaluate methods of collaboration between the two systems (Harding, 1975; Green, 1980; Richeport, 1984; Kilonzo & Simmons, 1998; Lambo, 1964; Airhihenbuwa & Harrison, 1993; Bodeker, 2001) but it is also important to acknowledge the difficulties (Heggenhougen & Gilson, 1997; Kaaya & Leshabari, 2002).

It is likely that dialogue, collaboration, research and shared care may be easier with herbalists than with entirely religious healers. Nevertheless, spiritual leaders and religious healers are important stakeholders in implementing a mental health strategy and can play a significant role in challenging stigma, enabling greater integration of people with mental health problems and in promoting mental health within the community, notably during times of transition or trauma.

Positive links and mutual respect between mental health professionals and spiritual leaders enable cross-referral, increased social support and increased opportunities for raising awareness of mental health issues and reducing discrimination. Ben-Tovim (1985) describes methods of integrating Western care with patient and family desires to continue to use traditional methods of treatment where possible.

Patients, who first consult traditional healers tend to arrive at a tertiary psychiatric service much later than those who first consult primary care. Experience from the WHO Pathways to Care multisite project in Nigeria suggests that attempts to incorporate traditional healers into the overall health care system must include efforts to improve their referral skills for severely ill patients who are not responding to their care (Gureje et al., 1995). There have been efforts to produce diagnostic algorithms for traditional healers to encourage them to refer all cases of psychosis and organic epilepsy to the specialist services (Saeed et al., 2000).

Any simultaneous consultation of both traditional and Western systems needs to be explicit and its implications understood. For example, there may be a risk of overdose if patients are given both Western antipsychotics and pharmacologically active herbal remedies. This is not an infrequent issue in psychiatric hospitals in low-income countries where the relatives may bring in a traditional medicine for the patient without the staff knowing until the patient starts to exhibit increasing side-effects of the Western remedy.

Implications for primary health care

Some authors argue that the whole notion of primary health care implies the recognition of the traditional or informal health system through which the community cares for the health of its members.

> The strategy of PHC requires the acceptance of the traditional system, the understanding of its ways, the improvement of quality of its performance, and its proper relationship with the formal systems. (Vargas, 1979)

At the Alma Ata conference, WHO made recommendations involving traditional practitioners and birth attendants.

> They are often part of the local community, culture, and traditions, and continue to have high social standing in many places, exerting considerable influence on local health practices. With the support of the formal health system, these indigenous practitioners can become important also in organising efforts to improve the health of the community. (WHO, 1978)

Since then several WHO–AFRO statements have focused on this issue. In 1984, the document AFR/RC24/R5/1984 urged States to prepare legislation to support traditional medicine, while in Namibia in 1999 and 2000, further statements were issued.

If traditional healers are to be considered as health providers in primary mental health care, however, the challenging task of defining the process and parameters for collaboration with orthodox services needs to be addressed (Kaaya & Leshabari, 2002). These include ethical issues, professional training and accreditation, conceptual frameworks for illness, causal models and treatment.

Kilonzo & Simmons (1998) report that, in Tanzania, traditional healers have demonstrated a willingness to participate in orthodox training programmes, showing a special interest in Tanzanian psychiatrists' approach to community mental health work and a willingness to share their knowledge and skills in the management of mentally ill people. In 1995 the traditional healers formed a professional association, and one of their objectives, laid down in their constitution, is that of encouraging collaboration between Western-trained doctors and traditional healers, and of increasing communication between these two sectors by meetings and seminars.

Implications for training

There is clearly value in educating traditional mental health practitioners better in the diagnosis of mental illness, thus ensuring the referral of severe cases to the orthodox system if they are not responding well to traditional treatments. Similarly, some countries are exploring the extent to which knowledge about traditional medicine could be taught as part of Western-based medical or health training (Kamla Tsey, 1997).

There is also scope for evaluating the extent to which traditional healers could operate a form of shared care with the orthodox professionals, so that, for example, a person with schizophrenia in a rural village far from the clinic, could be seen regularly and frequently by the traditional healer between visits to the clinic. The traditional healer could be given guidelines for detecting early symptoms of relapse and for prompt re-referral to the clinic.

Furthermore, since each primary care unit in a low-income country may be responsible for a population of 10,000 and thus have 1,000 people with depression and anxiety at any one time (on a conservative estimate), traditional healers may play a valuable role in assessing and managing these non-psychotic disorders, and could be given guidelines for onward referral of those above a certain threshold of severity, chronicity and disability.

Implications for research and development

It would be useful to have more research on the morbidity patterns in those who consult traditional healers, on the efficacy and side-effects of traditional medicines and approaches, and on the health, social and economic outcomes achieved. It would then be possible to evaluate health care systems where traditional healers were explicitly used in the care of people with mental disorders. An international information resource is needed, providing methodological guidance on clinical trial methodology in traditional medicine and a pharmacopoeia for traditional medicines. Priority must be given to an international effort to ensure the conservation, cultivation and sustainable harvesting of medicinal plants and their environments. The safety of herbal medicines must be given some priority. International research capacity in this field – for example, guidelines on safety, the training of scientists, traditional health practitioners, and those who dispense herbal medicines – needs to be addressed.

The WHO–AFRO strategy on traditional medicine has been reprinted as AFR/RC50/R3: it calls for Member States to carry out research on plants, promote their use, document practice and efficacy, and dedicate resources to strengthening their research capacity. Until now, priority diseases in this research effort have been HIV/AIDS and malaria, together with a focus on fertility and oral health. Malaysia has also established an extensive and coherent research agenda for traditional medicines, and a standing committee for Traditional and Complementary Medicine was established in 1999, together with a technical committee which is working to develop a national pharmacopoeia and an international information resource in traditional medicine. In view of the high proportion of mentally disordered people consulting traditional healers, mental health and mental illness are clearly essential topics to include in the above research agenda.

All health research should be guided by ethical principles, but the field of traditional medicine has a record of neglect and exploitation of customary knowledge holders. The view that traditional medicines are crude commodities to be exploited as leads for conventional drug development, is not ethical. It should be replaced by a holistic research strategy aiming to provide maximum benefits to local communities – one that would respect traditional health practitioners, their intellectual capital, and fully engage the communities concerned (Bodeker et al., 2001).

For clinical trials on herbal medicines, there should be full respect for the Helsinki Declaration (World Medical Association, 1964), and all protocols should be in full accord with WHO guidelines (WHO, 1991). Intellectual property rights relating to traditional health care knowledge should be respected, and there should also be development of equitable models of benefit sharing between customary knowledge holders and those responsible for the development of pharmacological compounds (Dutfield, 1999). Research databases should belong to the communities from which they have been generated.

RELIGIOUS GROUPS AND CHURCHES

As we have seen above, many traditional healers incorporate a religious element into their healing, to a greater or lesser degree. This section considers the contribution of religious groups and churches per se to the care and support of people with mental illness. In some countries, religious shrines may also function as hospitals for people with mental illness. All major religions, especially Islam, have played and still play an important role in caring for people with mental illness. This section uses Christianity as an example.

Within the Christian religion, one of the most dramatic stories of Jesus's healing ministry involves a severely mentally disturbed man (Luke 8, v. 26–36). Although Christians, like others, often fear mental illness, they have a history of offering help. Medieval monasteries offered food, clothing and herbal remedies to mentally ill people. The Bethlem Royal and the Tuke Hospitals in the UK both had Christian origins. Parish priests gave support and advice to relatives, and may also have been confidants and confessors to people suffering from mental illness.

Today churches generally offer practical help and encourage acceptance and understanding of people with a history of mental health problems. A 1999 Health Education Authority booklet in the UK (*Promoting Mental Health: The Role of Faith Communities – Jewish and Christian Perspectives*) built upon the investigative work of a group of Christian and Jewish people linked to the UK NGO – the National Schizophrenia Fellowship – who considered how to provide simple help for clergy and their congregations.

Rose (1996) found that people with mental health problems considered church groups to be the most helpful and sympathetic group after their immediate friends, placing them above their own families. Copsey (1997) found that religious communities played an important role, and that health and social services often overlook spiritual needs. Too often there was a taboo about any discussion of religious beliefs and needs in drawing up treatment and care plans. Religious concepts or practices were sometimes regarded as symptoms of mental illness.

Chaplains in mental health services play an important role in helping staff to understand a person's spiritual needs and religious practices, and are especially helpful in distinguishing religious customs and concepts from psychiatric symptoms. Chaplains liaise with local faith groups, and they may adapt services and prayer sessions to meet sufferers needs. Like their parish colleagues, they celebrate the sacraments, or take occasional offices like baptism or funerals. The sacrament of reconciliation (or confession) may be particularly helpful for some Roman Catholics or Anglicans, bringing its own comfort, support and release from guilt. Chaplains are a source of advice to parish clergy about supporting people with mental illness.

Faith in itself may be a source of comfort and support, especially in the belief of a loving God, who is always there and ready to listen, whatever happens. Prayer and meditation have been shown to bring positive mental health benefits, and may help to calm a disturbed person, though that may not always be suitable for people with acute symptoms, or who are highly disturbed. Reading the scriptures may be a source of help and support, or even provide a guide to healthy living. Belonging to a religious community offers acceptance, and the understanding of the importance of deeper feelings and longings. Taking doubts seriously and being prepared to listen may also be helpful to sufferers.

Although religious authority must be used carefully and wisely, priests, pastors, rabbis and imams may be able to persuade their members to receive treatment.

Churches and religious groups offer a wide range of help and services. In the UK, the Association for Pastoral Care in Mental Health trains local Christian volunteers as befrienders to people with mental health problems. Some religious orders of monks or nuns may run residential homes as well as being involved in providing time, help and support. Local churches or synagogues may run drop-in centres, clubs or even specialist day services for people with mental health problems. Counselling, pastoral visits, respite for carers, hospitality to sufferers, and non-therapeutic listening may all be offered under church auspices, but provision will vary from area to area. Carers also need practical and psychological support, and someone to listen patiently to their problems. Sympathetic fellow worshippers may have time to do this as a friend who knows and understands the family and their locality, without being a professional. Church membership brings opportunities for socialising and outings, as well as belonging to a community. It can assist people in relating or belonging to the wider local community, and even in taking advantage of its resources for help or leisure.

Clergy find that people with mental health problems are often drawn to churches, either to religious services or to seek individual help. As long as this is freely given in the light of helping a troubled individual who is a beloved child of God, this is likely to offer comfort and reassurance, but should not be used as a bargaining tool to obtain religious allegiance. Many congregations are quite patient in the face of strange behaviour and gestures which harm no one. If they see violence or fear for children's safety, or are regularly disturbed by disruptive shouting or abusive language, then they will try to eject the person. They need help in understanding strange behaviour and in knowing how to deal with disruptive outbursts.

The attitude of some charismatic or evangelical churches is unhelpful since they tend to regard mental illness as the result of wrong-doing or even demon possession. Their members may take a judgemental attitude and induce guilt. 'You're not praying enough'. Sometimes they resort to exorcism when in fact psychiatric advice and medication are needed. Exorcism may be very dramatic and frightening for a disturbed person, possibly playing into their delusional system rather than releasing them from their fear. Family members or carers may find themselves stigmatised, as well as being upset by their methods of exorcism. In the Roman Catholic and Anglican churches certain experienced priests are authorised by the Diocesan bishop to act as exorcists, and all other clergy or congregations have to refer to them. This provides good safeguards, and is unlikely to prevent psychiatric treatment being sought or encouraged when that is needed.

Some charismatic or evangelical groups believe it is their duty to proclaim and practise Christian joy, so there may be little sympathy for those who become depressed, failing to understand that depression may have an endogenous basis, rather than being a symptom of spiritual weakness. They may even discourage the person from going for treatment. The mental health chaplains should be able to advise on the nature of such groups if staff, users or relatives are concerned about their attitudes. Modern mental health care rightly stresses the importance of a holistic approach. It is important that all care staff are aware of the importance of recognising spiritual needs, and of drawing upon the goodwill of local faith groups in meeting those needs.

CHAPTER FOURTEEN

Tackling disaster and conflict and supporting refugees

Key Points

- *Disaster and conflict are widespread and common world wide.*
- *The potential impact on the mental health of the population is huge.*
- *This needs to be managed systematically through strategies for post-conflict reconstruction, prevention, developing responsive primary and secondary care, and through education.*

INTRODUCTION

More than 50 countries have experienced significant periods of conflict in the last two decades and peace-keeping operations alone cost the international community $3 billion in 1995. Although conflicts have happened in both rich and poor countries, they are relatively much more common in poor countries and 15 of the 20 poorest countries in the world have had a major conflict in the last 15 years. Conflicts have also spilled across the borders of neighbouring states and nearly every low-income country is adjacent to a country that has experienced breakdown and war. Conflicts in Africa as well as elsewhere have intensified the disinvestments in the education and health sectors, destroyed schools, displaced populations, reduced the numbers of teachers through death, displacement or mobilisation into the military, and greatly reduced planning and administrative capacity (Colletta et al., 1996).

The transition to peace is often characterised by insecurity, uncertainty and repeated cycles of violence before lasting solutions take hold. Thirty countries have had more than 10% of their population displaced through conflict and in ten countries the percentage is more than 40%. More than 90% of the casualties have been civilians. More than 100 million landmines have been laid, causing continuing casualties and blocking free movement, agriculture and economic development for many years after the conflict itself. Whole generations have grown up in cultures of armed

161

warfare and violence. The consequences of the conflict itself and the post-conflict aftermath for the mental health of the affected populations, and for the care of those who are already severely mentally ill, are enormous and devastating with ramifications for the capacity of the country to rebuild its assets, its social structures and its economic capacity.

The number of people of concern to the United Nations High Commissioner for Refugees rose from 17 million in 1991 to more than 27 million in 1995. Other estimates are much higher still (Instituto del Tercer Mundo, 1997). For many years, the refugee problems were considered as essentially African, South East Asian or Latin American. However, refugee movements have increased in the east and centre of Europe, the Caribbean, the Caucasus and the south of Asia, and many people only feel safe in refugee camps. The world's refugee burden is carried overwhelmingly by the poorest countries of the world. The 20 countries with the highest ratio of refugees have an annual per capita income average of 700 dollars (Instituto del Tercer Mundo,1997).

THE CONTRIBUTION TO DEATH, DISEASE AND DISABILITY

Violent conflict and the long-term dislocation of populations outrank natural disasters in the scale of death, disease and disability they cause. The social disorder is compounded by public health crises: epidemics of infectious diseases, malnutrition, widespread desperation and psycho-social disorders. Displaced people often suffer extraordinarily high mortality rates in the first few months of arriving in camps; mortality rates of 10 to 20 times higher than baseline are not uncommon. Most deaths in complex emergencies are caused by preventable or treatable diseases such as measles, tuberculosis, malaria and respiratory infections. It is not known how far rates of suicide are increased in such situations, or how far the presence of psycho-social disorder contributes to death from physical disorder in conflict and post-conflict situations. However, we do know that the presence of psycho-social disorders contributes to low compliance with vaccination programmes, nutrition, oral rehydration therapy and antibiotic therapy for TB. It also contributes to risky sexual behaviour, contributing to the spread of AIDS.

The inability to bury loved ones according to cultural mores

A great source of stress in many if not most cultures is the inability to bury loved ones according to their cultural mores. Some victims have had to witness the rotting corpses of loved ones, and have been unable to prevent the animal and enemy desecration of bodies. They usually lack the financial means to accommodate the care and feeding of mourners and are unable to gather enough mourners as the family may have perished or their whereabouts may be unknown. The remaining family members may be too traumatised and disoriented to participate, or the specific stages of the funeral rites may be too many and too complex to complete.

THE VULNERABILITY OF WOMEN AND CHILDREN

Women and children bear a particularly heavy burden in post-conflict situations. Many have witnessed the indiscriminate murder or torture of family and children, or have even been forced to participate in the killing and maiming of loved ones or members of other ethnic groups, as in Rwanda. Women may have been sexually assaulted, and experienced the stigma of rejection and avoidance, and perhaps become infected with sexually transmitted diseases or HIV. Some women are accused of collaboration with the enemy due to forced sexual alliances and some may have produced a child as a result of rape. In conflicts inspired by ethnic hatred, women may be rejected by their spouse and community because of their ethnic background, and they will experience feelings of guilt and distress if they have lost or abandoned their children. They often have to flee their home or place of refuge on more than one occasion and become impoverished by the frequent upheaval.

The dual burden on women

While both sexes are affected by emotional stress, mental illness, displacement and public insecurity, women in post-conflict situations often have to tend not only to their own needs but also to the needs of their family members. The special needs of women are often forgotten under the pressures of everyday living when each day is a fight for survival. The women tend to manage the household, look after the physical health needs and attend to the emotional needs of the family. In some communities, women rape victims are shunned by families and spouses for bearing children of the enemy, leading to considerable costs in social cohesion as well as damage to the parenting of existing and new children. Indeed, in some cultures, the tradition may be that a raped woman is to blame, and that family honour may only be preserved by her death. In such situations women may well wish to suppress their experiences of rape, and not seek help, and appropriate assistance will need to be very carefully considered. Psychological interventions will need to go hand in hand with appropriate physical interventions for victims of repeated rapes, sexually transmitted diseases, maiming physical injuries and psychological trauma, and will need to be sensitive to the complex interplay of culture, stratification, societal flexibility, class and ethnicity.

The impact of armed conflict on children

Armed conflict takes a terrible toll on the development of children, affecting their attitudes, relationships with family and peers, their moral values and their understanding of the world about them. Abduction and/or forced recruitment by the fighting factions often forces the vulnerable and the innocent to become part of the conflict as child soldiers, or as human shields and hostages, or as coerced sexual partners. In this situation, child rights are grossly and repeatedly violated, leading to traumatisation of the children and their families.

Children who participate in wars lose much of their social and cultural adaptation, and they cope with conflict and pain by defiance, violence and regressive behaviour. They may also continue to suffer from debilitating injuries. They generally do not conform to the normal social role assigned to children. The activities in which they were involved as combatants, the events they witnessed, and their consequent behaviour, can give the mistaken impression that those children are mature beyond their years when in fact they are merely traumatised.

Many cannot return home to resume life with their surviving relatives because they feel an incredible sense of guilt from actions committed or observed as soldiers, and indeed some of the former child soldiers are unwanted by their families because of their brutality during the war. Furthermore, responsible adults are often unable to cope with the rearing and emotional support needed by former child soldiers who suffer from guilt, post-traumatic stress disorder and inadequate social skills and behaviour patterns inappropriate to a peacetime environment. (Examples of projects working with children in the aftermath of political conflict in South Africa and the former Yugoslavia are included in Kalmanowitz & Lloyd, 1997.)

THE PSYCHO-SOCIAL ROLE OF HUMANITARIAN AND RELIEF AGENCIES

Displacement and the process of becoming a refugee leads to a loss of self-confidence and self-esteem, poverty through loss of the means of livelihood, and a breakdown of cultural values, dependency, idleness and redundancy. Refugees are often overcome by anxiety, fear, hyper-vigilance, worry and bad memories. There is a deep sense of helplessness and the risk of suicide is substantially increased. As well as the effects on individuals there are also the effects on the group as a whole. It is therefore vital that humanitarian and relief agencies are aware of these issues and develop population programmes which incorporate attention to psychological and social needs as well as physical needs.

Experience from earlier refugee crises suggests that it is important to build in psycho-social rehabilitation as an integral part of the overall programme of rapid health assessment, public health and nutritional surveillance, basic nutritional advice, ensuring a source of clean water, sanitation and vector control, establishing preparedness for epidemics (investigation, lab capacity, guidelines for epidemic control and case management), guidelines on immunisation, promoting essential drug management and advice on emergency relief items, promoting TB control, facilitating reproductive health guidelines, and preventing HIV and other sexually transmitted diseases. There will also be a need for assuring the continuing treatment and care of people with pre-existing severe mental illness who have been displaced by the crisis and separated from their normal source of health and social care.

PROBLEMS OF TIMING, NUMBERS AND ACCESS

Unlike natural disasters, wars are often protracted, with deaths mounting each year. Access to the most vulnerable populations is often restricted and landmines are a particular problem, impeding movement in post-conflict countries. Sometimes the sheer volume of refugees and their movements make practical arrangements very difficult. For example, in Macedonia during the Kosovo crisis, there were over 250,000 refugees and large transfers at short notice between camps as new refugees arrived, making psycho-social work very difficult during the initial phase (WHO, 2000). Sometimes people with severe mental illness, often abruptly discharged from mental hospital for their own safety, are among the refugees and need speedy access to continued support and treatment. Sometimes the relevant health care professionals are also among the refugees and can be speedily mobilised to play a key role. Access to local specialist services for refugees may be slow and hampered by bureaucracy, financing issues and other logistics; therefore, much treatment that would normally be done in hospital may need to be handled in the refugee camps.

MANAGEMENT OF PSYCHOLOGICAL
CONSEQUENCES OF DISASTER

Lima et al. (1988) argue for the importance of involving primary care teams in the management of the medium- and long-term psychological consequences of a disaster. Disasters are more likely to affect socio-economically disadvantaged populations who have little access to specialised mental health care. The role of the specialised mental health sector, where it exists, should relate to programme design, implementation and evaluation; to the training and education of the primary care worker; and to providing him or her with continuing support through consultation and supervision. In disaster prone countries, a small national disaster mental health team should develop a simple and well-structured educational and training package adjusted to the particular country. Once a disaster strikes, this team becomes responsible for training the mental health team local to the affected community. The local mental health team will then provide training and continuing support to the general health sector and to the front line primary care workers, other sectors of the disaster-relief operation, and the community. The trained primary care worker will in turn provide routine mental health care to victims, families and affected communities. The specialised mental health worker will remain available for evaluation and/or treatment of referred patients whose psychiatric problems are too complex to be handled at the primary care level. In such situations, cognitive-behavioural techniques appear to be the method of choice (Yule & Canterbury, 1994).

The proposed activities for the primary mental health care of disaster victims are detailed below.

Health promotion and primary prevention in disasters

- To develop educational activities with the community under threat of an impending disaster; to address frequent emotional problems such as denial or anxiety.
- To collaborate with programmes being developed by the general health sector or other sectors, integrating mental health into all the proposed activities.
- To co-ordinate the mental health activities with the other sectors in the community that will become active in the forthcoming disaster.
- To be familiar with the disaster relief system being developed, the health and community resources available, and the mechanisms for accessing these services.
- To develop community activities to foster solidarity and support to obtain a collective response to the disaster structure.

Secondary prevention

- To train the primary care workers to identify and manage victims who present emotional problems, including:
  - providing ventilation and emotional support
  - facilitating access to other health services or community resources as needed

  - involving the family and other support persons to manage the emotional problems, but with appropriate regard to cultural issues
  - supporting the professional health workers through supervision, consultation or referral with the specialised mental health worker.

Tertiary prevention

- To ensure that the primary health care worker maintains close collaboration with victims and affected families to promote their community adjustment, facilitating the utilisation of available resources.
- To ensure that the primary health care worker works with the community to facilitate the assimilation of displaced victims who have been relocated to this community.

Indeed, disasters have been seen as an opportunity for developing a decentralised primary health care system (Seboron et al.; Pucheu, 1985).

KEY ISSUES FOR CONSIDERATION IN FUTURE DISASTERS

- It is important to integrate any specialist mental health provision with primary care and NGO psycho-social provision in a synergistic way.
- It is essential to collect information about, and pay attention to, local customs, traditions, reactions and symptom patterns.
- It is essential for specialist mental health teams and for primary care teams and NGOs giving psycho-social support to co-operate as much as possible with families and with the social structure among the refugees. For example, where refugees come from the same village, this grouping may be the most important source of social support and the primary point of reference for the refugees.
- It is important to consider confidentiality in situations where interpreters may need to be used.

Disaster preparedness may include

- Collecting information about local resources and giving them to all organisations who will be involved in psycho-social and specialist mental health support.
- Co-ordination arrangements between the international humanitarian organisations and the local mental health, primary care and NGO services.
- Explicit co-operation and referral mechanisms, supported by meetings, supervision, outcome monitoring and training.

- Joint task-orientated training for collaborative organisations tackling, for example, sexual violence and its results, including physical and psychological trauma, pregnancy and sexually transmitted diseases – e.g. on supporting breastfeeding as the optimal way to nourish an infant and to protect against disease.
- Assembling framework of all assessments, interventions and activities that should be available for the refugees.
- Assembling framework for identifying target groups that need different kinds of intervention and support.
- Designing models for working with families and the existing social networks, and models for self-help.
- Considering the provision of free phones (to obtain information about relatives), recreational activities and visits outside the camps which all have a positive impact on mental health and psychological well-being.
- Preparing an essential drugs list, based on the WHO list, and organising commissioning and delivery of supplies and distribution to primary and secondary care and international NGOs, negotiating as necessary with the Ministry of Health. Use guidelines for treatment.

Medium- and long-term issues

- Training primary care and social services in mental health and psycho-social issues.
- Improving specialist services and creating community services.
- Reconciliation programmes (local and national) to encourage and support an open dialogue to allow grief reactions, mourning and to decrease hatred and revenge persisting through lifetimes and generations.
- Where there are long-term communities of refugees and internally displaced people, stimulating the development of self-help groups to organise 'common space' for teaching, children's activities (e.g. sports, art therapy, needlework, psychological support, theatre groups) and for women's group meetings.

POST-CONFLICT RECONSTRUCTION

Sustainable financing of health and education services in post-conflict countries is more difficult because of the relatively greater poverty of the populations. Severely constrained public resources generally exclude formal welfare/social programmes that are common in richer parts of the world. Therefore, promotion of informal, family, community and

NGO-based welfare programmes assume special importance. The social welfare of women also presents special issues in sub-Saharan Africa because traditional law may prevent widows or women, whose husbands have fled or are prisoners, from inheriting land.

The importance of education as a contributor to health

The central importance of education has not always been given adequate recognition. Although educational needs do not seem as urgent or salient as health needs in the immediate post-conflict situation, it is of critical importance for normal social development and is a major determinant of physical and psychological health. In particular, education, particularly of girls, lowers total fertility, lowers infant mortality rates and maternal mortality rates, raises the age of marriage and increases the use of contraceptives. The education of women also increases their use of medical services and improves household health behaviour, including nutrition and diet. This is what UNICEF has termed the 'Generational impact of educating girls' (UNICEF, 1999).

In some countries, the education system does not prepare students for the kinds of work that might be available in those countries, and the feeling among youth that life holds few prospects makes it much easier to recruit them as fighters. It is therefore crucial to develop programmes that will not only facilitate post-conflict reconstruction but will also lead to conflict prevention in the future and social cohesion. Special educational projects are likely to be needed for former child and teenage soldiers. All schools will need support to combat bullying, to be able to deliver support to traumatised children and children of traumatised adults, and to support children to regain a sense of personal and social identity that does not depend on intolerance of others.

In addition to these more recognised issues, education has other important functions in the contexts of conflict and post-conflict environments. UNICEF has suggested that, among its other functions, education plays a critical role in normalising the situation for the child and in minimising the psycho-social stresses experienced because of the sudden and violent destabilisation of the child's immediate family and social environment that results from emergencies. It is essential, in assisting children, to deal with their future more confidently and effectively, and this can be instrumental in making it possible for them to develop a peaceful society. Furthermore, educational activities that include parents and other community members can play an important role in rebuilding family and community cohesiveness.

Consequences of conflict or disaster for population sub-groups

Consequences of internal displacement or displacement to refugee camps for children

These include:

- Separation from the nuclear family.
- Disappearance of the extended family.
- Loss of sources of affection, protection and support.
- Uprooting from familiar surroundings and cultural environment.
- Loss of social safety nets.
- Loss of close personal contacts.
- Changes in functioning of the family where parents cease to be powerful.
- Impossibility of attending school.

Difficulties faced by children on arrival in a refugee camp, or new environment

These include:

- Discovering and integrating into a new community.
- Looking for parents and family members.
- Difficulties in going to school.
- Problems of social and cultural re-integration.
- Problems making new friends.
- Difficulties in finding food and clothing.
- Shifting to a new way of life geared to survival – becoming street children, or begging.
- Children taking responsibility for helping or replacing parents.

Consequences for displaced women

These include:

- Taking on the tasks of helping their husbands.
- Taking on the tasks of helping their own parents and their husband's parents and other members of both families.
- Dealing with the daily problems of finding food and water.
- Providing care and basic education for the children.

Consequences of war for women

These may be:

- Forced labour.

- Armed recruits.
- Sexual enslavement.
- Early marriage.

Consequences of displacement for adolescents and young men

These include:

- Socio-economic insecurity.
- Unemployment.
- Disintegration of the family unit.
- Involuntary divorce.
- Loss of cultural values.
- Loss of dignity and legitimacy.
- Rejection by their local community who no longer trust them.

CHAPTER FIFTEEN

Common problems with mental health strategies

IMPLEMENTING MENTAL HEALTH STRATEGIES

A number of common problems with mental health strategies are identified which need to be overcome if implementation is to be successful.

Lack of integration with overall health policy

At present, many countries are going through a process of health sector reform, but when the draft documents are examined, hardly any of them make more than a passing mention of mental health. This means that when the ministry finally comes to attend to mental health policy:

1. The policy is likely to be considered in an isolated fashion and will not articulate in an integrated way with physical health policy.
2. The available resources are likely to have been largely consumed for physical health.
3. Opportunities for concerted action favourable to both mental and physical health will be missed.

Lack of funding for community care

Research has shown that health and social outcomes are better where people are cared for in the community. Adequate care in the community is not cheaper than asylum care. However, many ministries of finance have seen de-institutionalisation as an opportunity to save money and have not made available appropriate funds for community care. This problem is exacerbated by the fact that it is impossible to close asylums until the last patient is in the community, and so double running costs are really needed to fund community care services while the asylum is still open. Governments are rarely willing to make such investment in mental health, and so the de-institutionalisation movement has tended to overburden the community health and social services which were not adequately prepared to receive them.

Lack of an adequate framework for care planning

There has frequently been a lack of attention to standards of health and social assessment, care planning, management, continuity of care and audit.

Lack of skills

There has not always been adequate basic and continuing skills-based training for the different members of the primary and secondary care teams to support them in the tasks they have to do (see page 139 on human resource strategies).

Lack of integration with the local culture and non-statutory sector

Policy often does not address the role of the non-statutory services; self-help groups, family support and traditional healers resulting in

- a lack of co-ordination;
- poor utilisation of the resources available;
- missed educational opportunities.

Lack of attention to the full range of illness

Policy often focuses exclusively on people with severe psychosis and does not pay attention to the heavy public health burden of depression. This results in a lack of attention to

- the role, structure and financing of primary care, and the way in which this influences the detection and care of people with mental illness;
- the interface between primary and secondary care;
- the adequate supply of essential medicines to primary care;
- adequate basic and continuing training in primary care.

Lack of machinery for monitoring the needs for care, the service inputs processes and outcomes

Policy often ignores the need for governments and local service providers to have a good system of monitoring mental health needs, services and health and social outcomes. Even the poorest of countries usually have helpful methods of monitoring physical disease but little attention is paid to mental health.

Lack of policy attention to health and social outcomes

An increasing number of countries are finding it helpful to set national and local targets to achieve specific health and social outcomes (Jenkins & Singh, 2000a). The fact that outcomes are difficult to measure on a routine basis has previously led to health service inputs and processes being used as proxy measures for outcomes, which of course they are not. The initial assumption was that 'service use = cure', and the amount of use equates with the severity of the condition, but it is now well recognised that use is not necessarily cure and that utilisation of services varies not only with socio-demographic factors, independent of the severity of symptoms and disability, but also with the characteristics of the service. Direct measures of health and social functioning have by far the strongest conceptual basis as relevant indicators of health outcome (Jenkins 1990, 1994).

Lack of evidence base

Countries frequently lack good epidemiological data, cost-effectiveness evidence and other health services research. There is often a lack of machinery to get this information directly to Ministers, policy-makers and the outside world.

Lack of involvement of service users and other stakeholders

> [Service users] provide a uniquely valuable perspective on services and it is impossible to get the best from a change process without actively involving them. (Department of Health, 1998)

Without user involvement in policy formulation and implementation at all levels, strategies may miss out in terms of

- meeting user needs;
- gaining support from the user movement;
- gaining user insights into service organisation and quality.

Services are, of course, there firstly for the user and secondly for society. Yet the views of the service users are often not heard or not taken into account. The reasons why the user voice is often ineffective include:

- Lack of access to background or strategic policy information, combined with the lack of resources to research alternative or additional information.
- Lack of knowledge of the legal and financial constraints under which services operate.

- Lack of clarity – or candour – as to what is available for discussion and what has already been decided.
- Unfamiliarity with the terminology (and jargon) employed in internal papers as well as government guidance and briefings.
- Nervousness about speaking up in meetings due to always being in a minority and being unused to formal meeting structures.
- Inability to set the agenda so that user reps are always in the position of responding to service proposals. Alternatively, lack of resources to develop proactive positional papers of their own.
- Lack of support outside of meetings.
- Lack of clarity in the planning process and, in particular, a failure of services to keep user reps informed of progress (or the lack of it) in the developments of proposals and the likely time-scales involved (McCulloch et al., 2000).

These problems can be addressed through a variety of means including:

- sensitive handling of meetings;
- multiple mental health service user representation;
- training for users;
- provision of papers in appropriate language;
- involvement from the beginning in shaping the consultation process;
- resourcing the user movement adequately.

Perverse incentives

The bureaucratic structures surrounding health and social care can often work against the mental health strategy. Common examples include:

1. Health and social care may be run by different political or administrative systems and have different finance streams. This can result in patients being shunted between sectors.
2. Boundaries between primary, secondary and tertiary care or between parts of the service (e.g. child and adolescent mental health services and adult services) can become so rigid that patients are either shunted around inappropriately or are lost to care.
3. Legal models that are poorly thought out and give too great an entitlement to certain groups to the detriment of others.
4. Different policies on issues such as IT, confidentiality, staff training, pay, complaints, etc., which impact on patients both indirectly and directly through poorly linked services.

Some of these issues are discussed in more detail in Chapters 3, 8 and 9.

Human rights treaties and other texts

International treaties on human rights

Universal Declaration of Human Rights (1948).

European Convention on Human Rights (Convention for the Protection of Human Rights and Fundamental Freedoms) (1950).

International Covenant on Civil and Political Rights (1966).

International Covenant on Economic, Social and Cultural Rights (1966).

International Convention on the Elimination of Racial Discrimination (1966).

Convention Against Torture and Other Inhuman or Degrading Treatment or Punishment (1984).

Convention on the Rights of the Child (1989).

Declaration on the Rights of Mentally Retarded Persons (Proclaimed by General Resolution 2856(XXVI) of 20 December 1971).

Principles of Medical Ethics relevant to the Role of Health Personnel, particularly Physicians, in the Protection of Prisoners and Detainees against Torture and Other Cruel, Inhuman or Degrading Treatment or Punishment (General Assembly Resolution 37/194 of 18 December 1982).

Body of Principles for the Protection of All Persons under Any Form of Detention or Imprisonment (General Assembly Resolution 43/173 of 9 December 1988).

Principles for the Protection of Persons with Mental Illnesses and the Improvement of Health Care (General Assembly Resolution 46/119 of 17 December 1991).

Relevant WHO documents on human rights and mental health legislation

Guidelines for the Promotion of Human Rights of Persons with Mental Disorders. World Health Organisation.

Mental Health Care Law: Ten Basic Principles. World Health Organisation, Geneva, 1996.

Draft Mental Health Act of Zanzibar (*and related amendments*). World Health Organisation, Geneva, October 1998.

Cases

X v. United Kingdom (European Court of Human Rights Judgments and Decisions, Series A, vol. 46 1981.

Winterwerp v. The Netherlands (European Court of Human Rights Judgments and Decisions, Series A, vol. 33 1979.

References

Abas, M., & Broadhead, J. (1997). Depression and anxiety among women in an urban setting in Zimbabwe. *Psychological Medicine, 27*, 59–71.

Abiodun, O.A. (1990). Mental health and primary care in Africa. *International Journal of Mental Health, 18*, 48–56.

Abiodun, O.A. (1991). Knowledge and attitudes concerning mental health of primary care workers in Nigeria. *The International Journal of Social Psychiatry, 37*, 113–120.

Acuda, S.W. (1983). Mental Health Problems in Kenya today: A review of research. *East African Medical Journal, 60*, 11–147.

Airhihenbuwa, C.O. & Harrison, I.E. (1993). Traditional medicine in Africa: Past present and future. In P. Conrad & E.B. Gallagher (Eds), *Health and Health Care in Developing Countries – Sociological perspectives*. pp. 122–133. Philadelphia: Temple University Press.

Alarcon, R.D., & Agnilar Gaxiola, S.A. (2000). Mental health policy development in Latin America. *Bulletin of WHO, 78*, 483–490.

Allgier (1993). *HIV/AIDS and Sex Education Strategies*. World Health Organisation.

Ammadeo, F., Gater, R., Goldberg, D., & Tansella, M. (1995). Affective and neurotic disorders in community based services: A comparative study in south Verona and south Manchester. *Acta Psychiatrica Scandinavica, 91*, 386–395.

Angermeyer, M.C. & Matschinger, H. (1996). The effect of personal experience with mental illness on the attitude towards individuals suffering from mental disorders. *Social Psychiatry and Psychiatric Epidemiology, 31*, 321–326.

Angus, J. & Murray, F. (1996). *Evaluation Frameworks: Criteria and methods in 'Arts for Health'*. London: King's Fund.

Armstrong, L. (1997). *The Primary Care Toolkit*. Department of Health, PO Box 410, Wetherby, LS23 7NL, UK.

Ashenden, R., Silagy, C., & Weller, D. (1997). A systematic review of effectiveness of promoting lifestyle change in general practice. *Family Practice, 14*, 160–175.

Asuni, T. (1979). The dilemma of traditional healing with special reference to Nigeria. *Social Science and Medicine, 138*, 33–39.

Asuni, T. (1986). Mental health in prison: The African perspective. *International Journal of Offender Therapy and Comparative Criminology, 30*, 1–9.

Asuni, T. (1990). Impact of research on designing strategies for preventing and treating dependence on drugs: The case for developing countries especially African countries. *Drug and Alcohol Dependence, 25*, 203–207.

Badger, L.W., Ackerson, B., Buttell, F., & Rand, E.H. (1997). The case for integration of social work psychosocial services into primary care practice. *Health and Social Work, 22*, 20–29.

179

Badger, L.W. & Rand, E.H. (1998). Unlearning psychiatry: A cohort effect. *International Journal of Psychiatry in Medicine, 18*, 123–135.

Barbee, J.G. (1998). Mixed symptoms and syndromes of anxiety and depression: Diagnostic, prognostic and etiologic issues. *Annals of Clinical Psychiatry, 10*, 15–29.

Barker, W., Anderson, R., & Chalmers, C. (1992). *Child Protection: The Impact of the Child Development Programme.* University of Bristol, Early Childhood Development Unit.

Barnes, M. & Shardlow, P. (1997). From passive recipient to active citizen: Participation in mental health user groups. *Journal of Mental Health, 6*, 289–300.

Barton, R. (1999). Psychosocial rehabilitation services in community support systems: A review of outcomes and policy recommendations. *Psychiatric Services, 50*, 525–534.

Baum, F. (2000). Social capital, economic capital and power: Further issues for a public health agenda. *Journal of Epidemiological Community Health, 54*, 409–410.

Beneduce, R. (1996). Mental disorders and traditional healing systems among the Dogon (Mali, West Africa). *Transcultural Psychiatry Research Review, 33*, 189– 220.

Ben-Tovim, D.I. (1983). A psychiatric service to the remote area of Botswana. *British Journal of Psychiatry, 142*, 199–203.

Ben-Tovim, D.I. (1985). Therapy managing in Botswana. *Australian and New Zealand Journal of Psychiatry, 19*, 88–91.

Berger, J.M. & Levin, S.M. (1993). Adolescents' substance abuse and HIV/AIDS: Linking the system. *Journal of Adolescent Clinical Dependency, 2*, 49–56.

Berrueta-Clement, J.R., Schweinhart, L.J., Barnett, W.S., Epstein, A.S., & Weikart, D.P. (1984). *Changed Lives: The Effects of the Perry Pre-school Program on Youth through Age 19.* High/Scope Educational Research Foundation, Monograph 8, High/Scope Press, Ypsilanti, USA.

Berry, H.L. & Rickwood, D.J. (2000). Measuring social capital at the individual level: Personal social capital, values and psychological distress. *International Journal of Mental Health Promotion, 2*, 35–44.

Berterame, S. (1994). Prevention of drug abuse among street children: Some lessons from UNDCP experience. *Meeting of WHO/PSA-IOGT on Street Children and Psychoactive Substances – Innovation and Cooperation.* Geneva, 18–22 April.

Bhugra, D., & Buchanan, A. (1993). Attitudes towards mental illness. In D. Bhugra & J. Leff (Eds). *Principles of Social Psychiatry.* London: Blackwell.

Bijl, R.V., van Zessan, G., & Rowelli, A. (1997). Psychiatric morbidity among adults in The Netherlands: The NEMESIS Study II Prevalence of Psychiatric Disorders. *The Netherlands Mental Health Survey and Incidence Study.* Ned Tijdschr Geneested. *December, 1997. 141(5)* 453–460.

Bindman, J., Johnson, S., Wright, S., Szmukler, G., Bebbington, P., Kuipers, E., & Thornicroft, G. (1997). Integration between primary and secondary services in the care of the severely mentally ill: Patients and general practitioners views. *British Journal of Psychiatry, 171*, 169–174.

Birchwood, M., McGorry, P., & Jackson, H. (1997). Early intervention in schizophrenia. *British Journal of Psychiatry, 170*, 2–5.

Black, D.R., Tobler, N.S., & Sciacca, J.P. (1998). Peer helping/involvement: An efficacious way to meet the challenge of reducing alcohol, tobacco and other drug use among youth: a meta analysis. *Journal of School Health, 68*, 87–93.

Bloch, M. (1991). Treatment of psychiatric patients in Tanzania. *Acta Psychiatrica Scandinavica, 83*, 122–128.

Bloom, B.L. (1985). *Stressful Life Event Theory and Research: Implications for Primary Prevention*, DHHS Publication No. ADM85-1385. Rockville: NIMH.

Bloom, B.L., Hodges, W.F., Kern, M.B., & McFaddin, S.D. (1985). A preventive intervention programme for the newly separated: Final evaluations. *American Journal of Orthopsychiatry*, *55*, 9–26.

Bobak, M., Hertzman, C., Skodova, Z., & Marmot, M. (1998). Association between psychosocial factors at work and non-fatal myocardial infarction in a population based case control study in Czech men. *Epidemiology*, 9, 43–47.

Bodeker, G. (2001). Lessons on integration from the developing world's experience. *British Medical Journal*, *322*, 164–167.

Bodeker, G., Jenkins, R., & Burford, G. (2001). International Conference on Health Research for Development (COHRED)., Bangkok, Thailand, 9–13 October 2000: Report on the Symposium on Traditional Medicine. *Journal of Alternative and Complementary Medicine*, *7*, 101–108.

Bond, G.R., Drake, R.E., Mueser, K.T., & Becker, D.R. (1997). An update on supported employment for people with severe mental illness. *Psychiatric Services*, *48*, 335–346.

Borrill, C.S., Wall, T.D., & West, M.A. et al. (1996). *Mental Health of the Workforce in NHS Trusts*. Universities of Sheffield and Leeds.

Bosma, H., Marmot, M.G., & Hemingway, H. (1997). Low job control and risk of coronary heart disease in Whitehall II (prospective cohort) study. *British Medical Journal*, *314*, 558–565.

Bosma, H., Schrijvers, C., & Mackenbach, J.P. (1999). Socioeconomic inequalities in mortality and importance of perceived control: Cohort study. *British Medical Journal*, *319*, 1469–1470.

Bosma, M. & Hosman, C. (1990). *Preventie op waarde geschat*. Nijmegen: Beta.

Brain, P.F. (1984). Human aggression and the physical environment. In Freeman (Ed.), *Mental Health and the Environment*, pp. 97–120. London: Churchill Livingstone.

Brown, J.S.L. & Cochrane, R. (1999). A comparison of people who are referred to a psychology service and those who self-refer to large-scale stress workshops open to the general public. *Journal of Mental Health*, *8*, 297–306.

Brown, J.S.L., Cochrane, R., & Hancox, T. (2000). Large-scale health promotion stress workshops for the general public: A controlled evaluation. *Behavioural and Cognitive Psychotherapy*, *28*, 139–151.

Brown, J.S.L., Cochrane, R., Mack, C.F., Leung, N., & Hancox, T. (1998). Comparison of effectiveness of large-scale stress management workshops with small stress/anxiety management training groups. *Behavioural and Cognitive Psychotherapy*, *26*, 219–235.

Brown, L. (1997). START: The arts in mental health. In C. Kaye & T. Blee (Eds), *The Arts in Health Care: A Palette of Possibilities*. London: Jessica Kingsley Publishers.

Brunner, E. & Marmot, M. (1999). Social organisation, stress and health. In M.G. Marmot & R.G. Wilkinson (Eds), *The Social Determinants of Health*. Oxford: Oxford University Press.

Bryson, J.M. (1995). *Strategic Planning for Public and Non-profit Organisations*. Jossey-Bass: San Francisco.

Burns, B.J., Regier, D.A., & Goldberg, I.G. et al. (1979). Future directions in primary care/mental health care research. *International Journal of Mental Health*.

Caan, W. (2000). Good for mental health: An academy for the social sciences. *Journal of Mental Health*, *9*, 117–119.

Caplan, G. (1961). *An Approach to Community Mental Health*. New York: Grune & Stratton.

Caplan, R.D., Proudfoot, J., Guest, D., & Carson, J. (1997). Effect of cognitive behavioural training on job finding among long term unemployed people. *Lancet*, *50*, 96–100.

Carstairs, G.M. (1973). Psychiatric problems of developing countries. *British Journal of Psychiatry, 123*, 271–277.

Caspe Healthcare Knowledge Systems (1998). *An Integrated Approach to Health at Work: Indicators of Good Practice – A Self-assessment Tool.* London: Health Education Authority.

Chaplin, R. (2000). Psychiatrists can cause stigma too. *British Journal of Psychiatry, 177*, 467.

Cheng, Y. & Kawachi, I. (2000). Association between psychosocial work characteristics and health functioning in American Women: Prospective study. *British Medical Journal, 320*, 1432–1436.

Clarke, G., Hawkins, W., Murphy, M., & Sheeber, L. et al. (1995). Targetted prevention of unipolar depressive disorder in an at risk sample of high school adolescents: A randomised trial of group cognitive intervention. *Journal of American Academy of Child and Adolescent Psychiatry, 34*, 312–321.

Cohen, S., Doyle, W.J., Skone, D.P., Rabin, B.S., & Gwaltney, J.M. (1997). Social ties and susceptibility to the common cold. *Journal of American Medical Association, 277*, 1940–1944.

Cohen, S. (Ed.), (1997). *Measuring Stress: A Guide for Health and Social Scientists.* Oxford: Oxford University Press.

Cohen, S., Tyrrell, D.A.J., & Smith, A.P. (1991). Psychological stress and susceptibility to the common cold. *New England Journal of Medicine* 325: 606–612.

Colgan, S., Bridges, K., & Faragher, B. (1997). A tentative START to community care. *Psychiatric Bulletin, 15*, 596–598.

Colletta, N.J., Kostner, M., & Wiedhofer, I. (1996). *The Transition from War to Peace in Sub-Saharan Africa.* Washington DC: The World Bank.

Commonwealth Department of Health and Aged Care (2000). *Promotion, Prevention and Early Intervention for Mental Health – A Monograph.* Mental Health and Special Programs Branch, Canberra.

Contributors to the Cochrane Collaboration and the Campbell Collaboration (2000). *Evidence from systematic reviews of research relevant to implementing the wider public health agenda.* NHS Centre for Reviews and Dissemination.

Cooper, H., Arber, S., Fee, L., & Ginn, J. (1999). *The Influence of Social Support and Social Capital on Health.* London: Health Education Authority.

Copsey, N. (1997). *Keeping Faith.* London: Sainsbury Centre for Mental Health.

Corney, R. (1992). The effectiveness of counselling in general practice. *International Review of Psychiatry, 4*, 331–338.

Corney, R. & Jenkins, R. (1992). *Counselling in General Practice.* London: Routledge.

Costello, E.J., Burns, B.J., Costello, A.J., Edelbrock, C., Dulcan, M., & Brent, D. (1988). Service utilisation and psychiatric diagnosis in paediatric primary care: The role of the gatekeeper. *Paediatrics, 82*, 435–441.

Countryside Commission (1997). *Public Attitudes to the Countryside.* Northampton.

Crisp, A.H., Gelder, M.G., & Rix, S. et al. (2000). Stigmatisation of people with mental illnesses. *British Journal of Psychiatry, 177*, 4–7.

Crowther, R., Bond, G., Huxley, P., & Marshall, M. (2000). Vocational rehabilitation for people with severe mental disorders (Protocol for a Cochrane Review). *The Cochrane Library*, Issue 3. Oxford.

Cuijpers, P. (1997). Bibliotherapy for unipolar depression: A meta-analysis. *Journal of Behaviour Therapy and Experimental Psychiatry, 28*, 139–147.

Curtis, T., Dellar, R., Leslie, E., & Watson, B. (2000). *Mad Pride: A Celebration of Mad Culture.* London: Spare Change Books.

Dalgard, O.S. & Tambs, K. (1997). Urban environment and mental health: A longitudinal study. *British Journal of Psychiatry*, *171*, 530–536.

Darbishire, L. & Glenister, D. (1998). *The Balance for Life Scheme: Mental health benefits of GP recommended exercise in relation to depression and anxiety*. Essex: University of Essex.

Davies, M. (Ed.), (2000). *The Blackwell Encyclopaedia of Social Work*. Oxford: Blackwell.

Dell, S. (1984). *Murder into Manslaughter*. Maudsley Monograph 27. Oxford University Press: Oxford, UK.

Department for Education and Employment (1999). *Sure Start: A Guide to Evidence-based Practice*. Nottingham: DFEE Publications.

Department of Health (1992). *The Health of the Nation*. London: Department of Health.

Department of Health (1994). *The Mental Illness Key Area Handbook*, 2nd edition. London: The Stationery Office.

Department of Health (1996a). *ABC of Mental Health: A Guide for Employers*. London: Department of Health.

Department of Health (1996b). *Building Bridges*. London: HMSO.

Department of Health (1998). *A First Class Service: Quality in the New NHS*. London: Department of Health.

Department of Health (1999a). *Our Healthier Nation: Saving Lives*. Cm 4386. London: The Stationery Office.

Department of Health (1999b). *National Confidential Inquiry into Suicide and Homicide by People with Mental Illness: Safer Services*. Leeds: Department of Health.

Department of Health (2000). *Attitudes to Mental Illness. RSGB Omnibus Survey*. Taylor Nelson Sofres plc.

Department of Health (2001). *Safety First: Five Year Report of the National Confidential Inquiry into Suicide and Homicide by People with Mental Illness*. London: Department of Health.

Desjarlais, R., Eisenberg, L., Good, B., & Kleinman, A. (1995). *World Mental Health: Problems and Priorities in Low Income Countries*. New York: OUP.

Dunn, S. (1999). *Creating Accepting Communities: Report of the MIND Inquiry into Social Exclusion and Mental Health Problems*. London: Mind Publications.

Durlak, J.A. (1995). *School Based Prevention Programs for Children and Adolescents*. California: Sage.

Durlak, J.A. & Wells, A.M. (1997). Primary prevention mental health programs for children and adolescents: A meta-analytic review. *American Journal of Community Psychology*, *25*, 115–152.

Dutfield, G. (1999). Rights, resources and responses. In D.A. Posey (Ed.), *Cultural and Spiritual Values of Biodiversity: A Complementary Contribution to the Global Biodiversity Assessment*. Nairobi: Intermediate Technology Publications and UN Environment Programme, pp. 503–546.

Edgerton, R.B. (1980). Traditional treatment for mental illness in Africa: A review. *Culture, Medicine and Psychiatry*, *4*, 167–189.

Eliany, M. & Rush, B. (1992). *How Effective are Alcohol and other Drug Prevention and Treatment Programmes? A Review of Evaluation Studies*. A Canada's Drug Strategy Baseline report. Health Promotion Studies Unit, Health Promotion Directorate, Health Services and Promotion Branch, Health and Welfare, Canada.

Ellison, C.G. & Levin, J.S (1998). The religion–health connection: Evidence, theory and future directions. *Health Education and Behaviour*, *25*, 700–720,

Emshof, J.G. (1990). A preventive intervention with children of alcoholics: protecting the children. *Prevention in Human Services*, 225–253.

Englund, H. (1998). Death, trauma and ritual: Mozambican refugees in Malawi. *Social Science and Medicine*, *46*, 1163–1174.

Ezeji, P.N. & Sarvela, P.D. (1992). Health care behaviour of the Ibo tribe of Nigeria. *Health Values*, *16*, 31–35.

Farrell, M., Howes, S., Taylor, C., Lewis, G., Jenkins, R., Bebbington, P., Jarvis, M., Brugha, T., Gill, B., & Meltzer, H. (1998). Substance misuse and psychiatric comorbidity: An overview of the OPCS surveys. *British Journal of Addiction*, *23*, 909–918.

Feingold, A. & Slammon, W.R. (1993). A model integrating mental health and primary care services for families with HIV. *General Hospital Psychiatry*, *15*, 290–300.

Felner, R.D. & Adan, A.M. (1988). The school transitional environment project: An ecological intervention and evaluation. In R.H. Price, E.L. Cowen, R.P. Lorian, & J. Ramos-McKay (Eds), *Fourteen Ounces of Prevention: A Casebook for Practitioners*. Washington: American Psychological Association.

Ferrie, J.E., Shipley, M.J., & Marmot, M. (1998). An uncertain future: The health effects of threats to employment security in white collar men and women. *American Journal of Public Health*, *88*, 1030–1036.

Foster, K., Meltzer, H., Gill, B., & Hinds, K. (1996). *OPCS Surveys of Psychiatric Morbidity in Great Britain*. Report No. 8: *Adults with a Psychotic Disorder Living in the Community*. London: The Stationery Office.

Friedli, L. (1999). From the margins to the mainstream: the public health potential of mental health promotion. *The International Journal of Mental Health Promotion*, *1*(2), 30–36.

Friedli, L. (2000a). Mental health promotion: Rethinking the evidence base. *The Mental Health Review*, *5*, 15–18.

Friedli, L. (2000b). A matter of faith: Religion and mental health. *International Journal of Mental Health Promotion*. *2*(2), 7–13.

Friedman, R., Sobel, D. et al. (1995). Behavioural medicine, clinical health psychology and cost offset. *Health Psychology*, *14*, 509–518.

Gallagher, E.B. (1993). Modernisation and medical care. In P. Conrad & E.B. Gallagher (Eds), *Health and Health Care in Developing Countries*, pp. 285–306. Philadelphia: Temple University Press.

Garssen, J., Abdul-Wakil, I., & Bondestan, S. (1988). *The Mental Health Programme in Zanzibar — Results of the 1998 Survey on Prevalence and Treatment of Mental Disorders and Epilepsy*. Zanzibar: Ministry of Health.

Gask, L., Rogers, A., Roland, M., & Morris, D. (2000). *Improving Quality in Primary Care: A Practical Guide to the National Service Framework for Mental Health*. National Primary Care Research & Development Centre.

Giel, R. (1978). Psychiatry in developing countries. *Annals of Psychiatry*, *8*, 315–320.

Giel, R. & Harding, T.W. (1976). Psychiatric priorities in developing countries. *British Journal of Psychiatry*, *128*, 513–522.

Gill, B., Meltzer, H., Hinds, K. & Petticrew, M. (1996). *OPCS Surveys of Psychiatric Morbidity in Great Britain*; Report No. 7: *Psychiatric Morbidity among Homeless People*. London: The Stationery Office.

Global Forum for Health Research (2000). *10/90 Report on Health Research 2000*. Geneva: Global Forum for Health Research. http: //www.globalforumhealth.org/report.htm

Glover, G. & Gould, K. (1996). Performance indicators in mental health services. In Thornicroft and Strathdee (Eds), *Commissioning Mental Health Services*. London: HMSO, pp. 265–272.

Goffman, E. (1961). *Asylums: Essays on the Social Situation of Mental Patients and other Inmates*. Harmondsworth: Penguin.

Goldberg, D.P., Gater, R., Sartorius, N., Ustun, T.B., Piccinelli, M., Gureje, O., & Rutter, C. (1997). The validity of two versions of the GHQ in the WHO study of mental illness in general health care. *Psychological Medicine, 27,* 191–197.

Goldberg, D.P. & Huxley, P. (1992). *Common Mental Disorders – A Biopsychosocial Model.* London: Routledge & Kegan Paul.

Goldberg, D. & Gourney, K. (2000). *The General Practitioner, the Psychiatrist and the Burden of Mental Health Care.* Maudsley Discussion Paper. Institute of Psychiatry, King's College, London.

Goodwin, J.S. (2000). Glass half full attitude promotes health in old age. *Journal of the American Geriatrics Society, 48,* 473–478.

Gournay, K. & Brooking, J. (1995). The community psychiatric nurse in primary care: An economic analysis. *Journal of Advanced Nursing, 22,* 768–778.

Gowan, N. (1999). *Healthy Neighbourhoods.* London: King's Fund.

Grant, T. (2000). *Physical Activity and Mental Health: National Consensus Statements and Guidelines for Practice.* London: Somerset Health Authority/Health Education Authority.

Green, E.C. (1980). Roles for African traditional healers in mental health care. *Medical Anthropology, 4,* 489–522.

Griffiths, S., Wylie, I., & Jenkins, R. (1992). *Creating a Common Profile.* London: HMSO.

Gureje, D. & Alem, A. (2000). Mental health policy developments in Africa. *Bulletin of WHO, 78,* 475–482.

Gureje, O., Acha, R.A., & Odeide, A. (1995). Pathways to psychiatric care in Ibadon, Nigeria. *Tropical and Geographical Medicine, 47,* 125–129.

Harding, T. (1975). Traditional healing methods for mental disorders. *WHO Chronicle, 31,* 436–440.

Harding, T.W., de Arango, M.V., Baltazar, J. et al. (1980). Mental disorders in primary health care: A study of their frequency in four developing countries. *Psychological Medicine, 10,* 231–241.

Harpham, T. (1994). Urbanisation and mental health in developing countries: A research role for social scientists, public health professionals and social psychiatrists. *Social Science and Medicine, 39,* 233–245.

Harris, E.C. & Barraclough, B. (1998). Excess mortality of mental disorder. *British Journal of Psychiatry, 173,* 11–53.

Harris, E. & Willis, J. (1997). Developing healthy local communities at local government level: Lessons from the past decade. *Australian and New Zealand Journal of Public Health, 21,* 4.

HEA (1997). *Mental Health Promotion: A Quality Framework.* London: Health Education Authority.

HEA (1998b). *Effectiveness of Health Promotion Interventions in the Workplace: A Review.* London: Health Education Authority.

HEA (1998c). *Living with Schizophrenia.* London: Health Education Authority.

HEA (1999a). *Community Action for Mental Health.* London: Health Education Authority.

HEA (1999b). *Promoting Mental Health: The Role of Faith Communities – Jewish and Christian Perspectives.* London: Health Education Authority.

HEA (2000). *Art for Health: A Review of Good Practice in Community Based Arts Projects and Interventions which Impact on Health and Well-being.* London: Health Education Authority.

Health and Safety Commission (1999). *Managing Stress at Work.* Discussion Document, DDE10.

Health and Safety Executive (1998). *Managing Work Related Stress – A Guide for Managers and Teachers in Schools*. Suffolk: HSE Books.

Heaney, C.A. (1992). Enhancing social support at the workplace: Assessing the effects of the Caregiver Support Programme. *Health Education Quarterly, 18*, 477–494.

Heaney, C., Price, R., & Rafferty, J. (1995). Increasing coping resources at work: A field experiment to increase social support, improve work team functioning and enhance employee mental health. *Journal of Organisational Behaviour, 16*, 335–352.

Heaver, R. (1995). *Managing Primary Health Care – Implications of the Health Transition*. World Bank Discussion Paper 276. Washington: The World Bank.

Hecht, R. (1995). Urban health – an emerging priority for the World Bank. In T. Harpham and M. Tanner (Eds), *Urban Health in Developing Countries – Progress and Prospects,*, pp. 123–141. New York: St Martin's Press.

Heggenhougen, K.H. & Gilson, L. (1998). Perceptions of efficacy and the use of traditional medicine with examples from Tanzania. *Curare, 20*, 5–13.

Heijmens Visser, J., van der Ende, J., Koot, H.M., & Verhulst, F.C. (2000). Predictors of psychopathology in young adults referred to mental health services in childhood or adolescence. *British Journal of Psychiatry, 177*, 59–65.

Henderson, A.S. (1986). Epidemiology of mental illness. In H. Hafner, G. Moschel, & N. Sartorius (Eds), *Mental Health of the Elderly: A Review of the Present State of Research*. Berlin: Springer.

Henderson, G. & McCollam, A. (2000). Using a wider lens – focusing on social inclusion. *The Mental Health Review, 5*, 30–32.

Henk, M.L. (1989). *Social work in primary care*. Newbury Park, CA: Sage.

Herrmann, C., Brand-Driehorst, S. et al. (1998). Diagnostic groups and depressed mood as predictors of 22 month mortality in medical inpatients. *Psychosomatic Medicine, 60*, 570–577.

Hersey, J.C., Kilnamoff, L.S., Lam, D.J., & Taylor, R.L. (1984). Promoting social support: The impact of California's 'friends can be good medicine' campaign. *Health Education Quarterly, 11*, 293–311.

Hillert, A., Sandmann, J., Ehmig, S.C. et al. (1999). The general public's cognitive and emotional perception of mental illnesses: An alternative to attitude research. In J. Guimon, W. Fischer, & N. Sartorius (Eds), *The Image of Madness: The Public Facing Mental Illness and Psychiatric Treatment*, Basel: Karger.

Hindley, P. (1997). Psychiatric aspects of hearing impairments. *Journal of Child Psychology and Psychiatry* 38, 101–117.

Hippisley-Cox J., Fielding, K., & Pringle, M. (1998). Depression as a risk factor for ischaemic heart disease in men: Population based case control study. *British Medical Journal, 316*, 1714–1719.

Hodnett, E.D. (2000). Support during pregnancy for women at increased risk. *Cochrane Review: The Cochrane Library*, Issue 1, Oxford.

Hodnett, E.D. & Roberts, I. (2000). Home based social support for socially disadvantaged mothers. *Cochrane Review: The Cochrane Library*, Issue 3. Oxford: Update Software.

Hoggett, P., Stewart, M., Razzaque, K., & Barker, I. (1999). *Urban Regeneration and mental Health in London*. London: King's Fund.

Hosman, C. & Veltman, N. (1994). *Prevention in Mental Health: A Review of the Effectiveness of Health Education and Health Promotion*. Utrecht: Landelijk Centrum GVO.

Hoult, J. & Reynolds, I. (1988). Schizophrenia: A comparative trial of community orientated and hospital orientated care. *Acta Psychiatrica Scandinavica, 69*, 359–372.

Huxley, P. (1997). *Arts of prescription: An evaluation*. A report to Stockport Leisure Services (Stockport Metropolitan Borough, Romiley) and the Health Promotion Department of Stockport Health Care NHS Trust.

Instituto del Tercer Mundo (1997). *The World Guide 1997/8*. Oxford: New Internationalist Publications Ltd.

International Union for Health Promotion and Education (1999). *The Evidence of Health Promotion Effectiveness: Shaping Public Health in a New Europe*. Brussels and Luxembourg: European Commission.

Jablensky, A. (1986). Epidemiology of schizophrenia: A European perspective. *Schizophrenia Bulletin, 12*, 52–73.

Jablensky, A. (1987). Multi-cultural studies and the nature of schizophrenia: A review. *Journal of the Royal Society of Medicine, 80*, 612–617.

Jablensky, A. (2001). Schizophrenia. In *Psychiatric and Neurological Disorders in Low Income Countries*. Washington: Institute of Medicine.

Jablensky, A., Korten, A., Ernberg, G., Anker, M., Cooper, J.E., & Day, R. (1986). Manifestations and first contact incidence of schizophrenia in different cultures. *Psychological Medicine, 16*, 909–928.

Jablensky, A., Sartorius, N., Ensberg, G., Anker, M., Korten, A., Cooper, J.F., Day, R., & Bertelsen, A. (1992). Schizophrenia: Manifestations, incidence and cause in different cultures – A World Health Organisation ten country study. *Psychological Medicine Monograph, Suppl. 20*: 1–97.

Jackson, C. & Birchwood, M. (1996). Early intervention in psychosis: Opportunities for secondary prevention. *British Journal of Clinical Psychology, 55*, 487–502.

Janzen, J.M. (1978). *The Quest for Therapy. Medical Pluralism in Lower Zaire*. Berkeley: University of California Press.

Jayerba, D.A. (1988). Notes on the utilisation of traditional and modern/western mental health practices among the Yoruba, Nigeria. *International Journal of Nursing Studies, 25*, 179–184.

Jenkins, R. (1985a). Sex differences in minor psychiatric morbidity. *Psychological Medicine Monograph No. 7*. Cambridge University Press: Cambridge.

Jenkins, R. (1985b). Minor psychiatric morbidity in civil servants and its contribution to sickness absence. *British Journal of Industrial Medicine, 42*, 147–154.

Jenkins, R. (1985c). Minor psychiatric morbidity and labour turnover. *British Journal of Industrial Medicine, 42*, 534–539.

Jenkins, R. (1990). Towards a system of outcome indicators for mental health care. *British Journal of Psychiatry, 157*, 500–514.

Jenkins, R. (1992). Developments in primary care of mental illness – a forward look. *International Review of Psychiatry, 4*, 237–242.

Jenkins, R. (1994). Ageing in learning difficulties: The development of health care outcome indicators. *Journal of Intellectual Disability Research, 38*, 257–264.

Jenkins, R. (1997). Reducing the burden of mental illness. *Lancet, 349*, 1340.

Jenkins, R. (1998a). Mental health and primary care-implications for policy. *International Review of Psychiatry, 10*, 158–160.

Jenkins, R. (1998b). Linking epidemiology and disability measurement with mental health service policy and planning. *Epidemiologia Psichiatria Sociale, 7*, 120–126.

Jenkins, R. (2001a). Depression. In *Psychiatric and Neurological Disorders in Low Income Countries*. Washington: Institute of Medicine.

Jenkins, R. (2001b). Making psychiatric epidemiology useful: The contribution of epidemiology to government policy. *Acta Psychiatrica Scandinavica, 103*, 2–14.

Jenkins, R. (2001c). World Mental Health Day: Social Psychiatry and Psychiatric Epidemiology.

Jenkins, R., Bebbington, P., Brugha, T., Farrell, M., Gill, B., Lewis, G., Meltzer, H., & Petticrew, M. (1997a). The national psychiatric morbidity surveys of Great Britain. *Psychological Medicine, 27*, 765–774.

Jenkins, R., Bebbington, P., Brugha, T., Farrell, M., Gill, B., Lewis, G., Meltzer, H., & Petticrew, M. (1997b). The national psychiatric morbidity surveys of Great Britain – Initial findings for the Household Survey. *Psychological Medicine, 27*, 775–791.

Jenkins, R., Bebbington, P., Brugha, T., Farrell, M., Gill, B., Lewis, G., Meltzer, H., & Petticrew, M. (1998a). British Psychiatric Morbidity Survey. *British Journal of Psychiatry, 173*, 4–7.

Jenkins, R., Kessler, R., Leaf, P., & Scott, J. (2000). Systems of psychiatric care – principles and Desiderata of good services. In H. Helmchen, F. Henn, H. Laurer, & N. Sartorius (Eds), *Psychiatrieder Gegenwart*, Vol. 11, Chap. 11. Heidelburg: Springer-Verlag.

Jenkins, R. & Knapp, M. (1996). Use of health economic data by health administrations in national health systems. In M. Moscarelli, A. Rupp, & N. Sartorius (Eds), *The Handbook of Mental Health Economics and Health Policy*, Vol. 1. *Schizophrenia*. Chichester: Wiley.

Jenkins, R., Mussa, M., & Saidi, S. (1998b). *The National Mental Health Plan for Zanzibar*. London: WHO Collaborating Centre.

Jenkins, R. & Singh, B. (1999). National suicide prevention strategies. *Psychiatric ?*, 9–30.

Jenkins, R. & Singh, B. (2000a). Measuring outcomes in mental health-implications for policy. In G. Thornicroft (Ed.), *Measuring Outcomes for Mental Health*. Cambridge University Press: Cambridge.

Jenkins, R. & Singh, B. (2000b). Health targets. In G. Thornicroft, T. Brewin, & J. Wing (Eds), *Measuring Mental Health Needs*. 2nd edition. Cambridge University Press: Cambridge.

Jenkins, R. & Singh, B. (2000c). Policy and practice in suicide prevention. *British Journal of Forensic Practice, 2*(1), 3–11.

Jenkins, R. & Singh, B. (2000d). General population strategies of suicide prevention. In K. Hawton & K. van Heeringen (Eds), *The International Handbook of Suicide and Attempted Suicide*, pp. 597–615. Chichester: Wiley.

Jenkins, R. & Strathdee, G. (2000). The integration of mental health care with primary care. *International Journal of Law and Mental Health, 238*, 277–291.

Jenkins, R. & Ustun, T.B. (1997). *Promoting Mental Health and Preventing Mental Illness in Primary Care*. Chichester: Wiley.

Jenkins, R. & Warman, D. (1993). *Promoting Mental Health Policies in the Workplace*. London: HMSO.

Johnson, J.V., Stewart, W., Hall, E.M., Fredlund, P., & Theorell, T. (1996). Long term psychosocial work environment and cardiovascular mortality among Swedish men. *American Journal of Public Health, 86*, 324–331.

Johnson, S., Thornicroft, G., Phelan, M., & Slade, M. (1996). Assessing needs for mental health services. In M. Tansella & G. Thornicroft (Eds), *Mental Health Outcome Measures*, 2nd edition. London: Gaskill.

Johnson, Z., Howell, F., & Molloy, B. (1993). Community mothers programme: Randomised controlled trial of non-professional intervention in parenting. *British Medical Journal, 306*, 1449–1452.

Johnstone, E. (1998). Diagnosis and classification. In *Companion to Psychiatric Studies*. Edinburgh: Churchill Livingstone, pp. 265–280.

Jonas, B.S., & Mussolino, M.E. (2000). Symptoms of depression as a prospective risk factor for stroke, *Psychosomatic Medicine, 62*, 463–472.

Jones, W.H.S. (1972). *Works of Hippocrates*, Vol. 1. Loeb Classical Library. London: Heinemann.

Joop de Jong (1996). A comprehensive public mental health programme in Guinea-Bissau: A useful model for African, Asian and Latin American countries. *Psychological Medicine, 26*, 97–108.

Jorm, A.F. (2000). Mental health literacy: Public knowledge and beliefs about mental disorder. *British Journal of Psychiatry*, *177*, 396–401.

Kaaya, S.F. & Leshabari, M.T. (2002). Depressive illness and primary health care in sub-Saharan Africa: with special reference to Tanzania. In *Health and Social Change in East Africa*. Dar es Salaam: Dar es Salaam University Press.

Kalmanowitz, D. & Lloyd, B. (1997). *The Portable Studio: Art Therapy and Political Conflict. Initiatives in Former Yugoslavia and South Africa*. London: Health Education Authority.

Kamla Tsey (1997). Traditional medicine in contemporary Ghana: A public policy analysis. *Social Science Medicine*, *45*, 1065–1074.

Kawachi, I., Kennedy, B.P., & Lochner, K. (1997a). Long live community: Social capital as public health. *The American Prospect*, *35*, 55–59.

Kawachi, I., Kennedy, B., et al. (1997b). Social capital, income inequality and mortality. *American Journal of Public Health*, *87*, 491–498.

Kawachi, I. & Kennedy, B.P. (1999). Income inequality and health: Pathways and mechanisms. *Health Services Research*, *34*, 215.

Kawachi, I., Kennedy, B.P., & Wilkinson, R.G. (1999). Crime: Social disorganisation and relative deprivation. *Social Science and Medicine*, *48*, 719.

Kempinski, R. (1991). Mental health and primary health care in Tanzania. *Acta Psychiatrica Scandinavica*, *83*, 112–121.

Kendrick, T., Sibbald, B., Burns, T., & Freeling, P. (1991). Role of general practitioners in care of long term mentally ill patients. *British Medical Journal*, *302*, 508–510.

Kessler, R.C., McGonagle, K.A., Zhaos, S. et al. (1994). Lifetime and 12 month prevalence of DSM IIIR psychiatric disorders in the United States – results from the National Comorbidity Study. *Archives of General Psychiatry*, *51*, 8–19.

Kilonzo, G.P. (1992). The challenges of rehabilitation psychiatry – the Tanzania experience. *Medicus – Magazine of the Kenyan Medical Association*, *11*, 6.

Kilonzo, G.P. (1998). *Drug demand reduction – an African overview*. Paper presented at the International Seminar on Drug Law Enforcement Agency, Arusha, 17–18 September.

Kilonzo, G.P. & Simmons, N. (1998). Development of mental health services for Tanzania: A reappraisal for the future. *Social Science and Medicine*, 419–428.

Kingdon, D. & Jenkins, R. (1996). Adult mental health policy. In G. Thornicroft & G. Strathdee (Eds), *Commissioning Mental Health Services*, pp. 1–12. London: HMSO.

King's Fund (2000). *Regeneration and Mental Health*. Briefing 3.

Kleinman, A. (1980). *Patients and Healers in the Context of Culture – an Exploration of the Borderland between Anthropology, Medicine and Psychiatry*. Berkeley: University of California Press.

Kulhara, P. (1994). Outcome of schizophrenia: Some transcultural observations with particular reference to developing country. *European Archives of Psychiatry and Clinical Neuroscience*, *244*, 227–235.

Lader, D., Singleton, N., & Meltzer, H. (2000). *Psychiatric morbidity among young offenders in England and Wales*. London: Office for National Statistics.

Lambo, T.A. (1964). The village of Aro. *Lancet*, *2 (7358)*, 513–514.

Lambo, T.A. (1965). Psychiatry in the tropics. *Lancet*, *2 (7422)*, 1119–1121.

Lambo, T.A. (1971). The right to health. *Nursing Journal of India*, *65*, 319.

Lambo, T.A. (1996). Socioeconomic change, population explosion and the changing phases of mental health programs in developing countries. *American Journal of Orthopsychiatry*, *26*, 77–83.

Lavaikainen, J., Lahtinen, E., & Lehtinen, V. (2001). *Public Health Approach on Mental Health in Europe*. Helsinki: National Research and Development Centre for Welfare and Health, STAKES. Ministry of Social Affairs and Health.

Lechat, M.E. (1979). Disasters and public health. *Bulletin of the World Health Organisation*, *57*, 11–17.

Ledermann, S. (1956). *Alcool. Alcolisme, Alcoholisation*. Paris: Presses Universitaires de Paris.

Lee, S. (1996). Reconsidering the status of anorexia nervosa as a Western culture bound syndrome. *Social Science and Medicine*, *42*, 221–234.

Lee, S. & Lee, A. (2000). Disordered eating in three communities of China: A comparative study of female high school students in Hong Kong, Shenzen and rural Hunan. *International Journal of Eating Disorders*, *27*, 317–327.

Leff, J. (2000). Transcultural psychiatry. In H.G. Gelder, J.L. Lopez-Ibor, & N. Andreason (Eds), *Textbook of Psychiatry*, pp. 12–15. London: Oxford University Press.

Levin, S. (1993). Public health care perspectives for the 1990s: What are the options? *Journal of Adolescent Chemical Dependency*, *2(3/4)*, 37–48.

Lewis, A.J. (1953). Health as a social concept. *British Journal of Sociology*, *4*, 109–124.

Lewis, G. & Booth, M. (1994). Are cities bad for your mental health? *Psychological Medicine*, *24*, 913–915.

Lewis, G., Bebbington, P., Brugha, T., Farrell, M., Gill, B., Jenkins, R., & Meltzer, H. (1998). Socioeconomic status, standard of living and neurotic disorder. *Lancet*, *352*, 605–609.

Lima, R.R., Santaonz, H., Lazano, J., & Lima, J. (1988). Planning for health/mental health integration in emergencies. In M. Lystad (Ed.), *Mental Health Response to Mass Emergencies – Theory and Practice. Psychosocial Stress Services No 12*. New York: Brunner/Mazel.

Link, B., Phelan, J., Bresnahan, M., Stueve, A., & Pescosolido, B.A. (1999). Public conceptions of mental illness: Labels, causes, dangerousness and social distance. *American Journal of Public Health*, *89*, 1328–1333.

Link, B., Struening, E., Rahav, M., Phelan, J., & Nuttbrock, L. (1997). On stigma and its consequences: Evidence from a longitudinal study of men with dual diagnoses of mental illness and substance abuse. *Journal of Health and Social Behaviour*, *38*, 177–190.

Lister-Sharp, D., Chapman, S., Stewart-Brown, S., & Sowden, A. (1999). *Health Promoting Schools and Health Promotion in Schools: Two Systematic Reviews*. London: Health Technology Assessment, No. 22.

Lloyd, K. & Jenkins, R. (1995). Primary care. In E. Paykel & R. Jenkins (Eds), *Prevention in Psychiatry*, pp. 198–209. London: Gaskell.

Lloyd, K., Jenkins, R., & Mann, A. (1996). The long term outcome of patients with neurotic illness in in general practice. *British Medical Journal*, *313*, 26–28.

Lock, K. (2000). Health impact assessment. *British Medical Journal*, *320*, 1395–1398.

Lynch, J., Due, P., Muntaner, C. et al. (2000). Social capital – is it a good investment strategy for public health? *Journal of Epidemiological Community Health*, *54*, 404–408.

Lystad, M. (1988). *Mental Health Response to Mass Emergencies – Theory and Practice*. New York: Brunner/Mazel.

MacLachlan, M. (1993a). Sustaining health service development in the Third World. *Journal of Royal Society of Health*, *113*, 132–133.

MacLachlan, M. (1993b). Mental health in Malaus – which way forward. *Journal of Mental Health*, *2*, 271–274.

Mann, A.H., Blizzard, R., Murray, J., Smith, J.A., Botega, N., & Wilkinson, G. (1998). An evaluation of practice nurses working with general practitioners to treat people with depression. *British Journal of General Practice*, *48*, 875–879.

Mann, A.H., Jenkins, R., & Belsey, E. (1981). The twelve-month outcome of patients with neurotic illness in general practice. *Psychological Medicine, 11*, 535–550.

Markman, H.J., Floyd, F.J., Stanley, S.M., & Storaasli, R.D. (1988 and follow up). Prevention of marital distress: A longitudinal investigation. *Journal of Consulting and Clinical Psychology, 56*, 210.

Marmot, M., Davey-Smith, G., Stansfield, S., Patel, C., et al. (1991). Health inequalities among British Civil Servants: The Whitehall II study. *Lancet, 337*, 1387–1393.

Marmot, M. & Wilkinson, R. (1999). *Social Determinants of Health*. Oxford: Oxford University Press.

Martin-Baro, I. (1994). *Writings for a Liberation Psychology*. Cambridge, Mass: Harvard University Press.

Marucha, P.T., Kiecolt-Glaser, J.K., & Favagehi, M. (1998). Mucosal wound healing is impaired by examination stress. *Psychosomatic Medicine, 60*, 362–365.

Matarasso, F. (1997). *Use or Ornament. The Social Impact of Participation in the Arts*. Stroud: Comedia.

Mavreas, V., Beis, A., Mouijias, A., Rigeni, F., & Lykersas, G. (1986). Prevalence of psychiatric disorders in Athens: A community study. *Social Psychiatry, 21*, 172–181.

McCulloch, A., Warner, L., & Villeneau, L. (2000). *Taking your Partners*. London: Sainsbury Centre for Mental Health.

McGorry, P.D. & Jackson, H.J. (1999). *The Recognition and Management of Early Psychosis: A Preventive Approach*. Cambridge: Cambridge University Press.

McKay, D. (2000). Stigmatising pharmaceutical advertisements. *British Journal of Psychiatry, 177*, 467–468.

Meltzer, H., Gill, B., Petticrew, M., & Hinds, K. (1995a). Report No. 1. *The prevalence of psychiatric morbidity among adults living in private households. OPCS Surveys of Psychiatric Morbidity in Great Britain*. London: The Stationery Office.

Meltzer, H., Gill, B., Petticrew, M., & Hinds, K. (1995b). Report No. 2, Physical complaints, service use and treatment of adults with psychiatric disorders. *OPCS Surveys of Psychiatric Morbidity in Great Britain*. London: The Stationery Office.

Meltzer, H., Gill, B., Petticrew, M., & Hinds. K. (1995c). Report No. 3, Economic activity and social functioning of adults with psychiatric disorders. *OPCS Surveys of Psychiatric Morbidity in Great Britain*. London: The Stationery Office.

Meltzer, H., Gill, B., Petticrew, M., & Hinds, K. (1996a). Report No. 4, The prevalence of psychiatric morbidity among adults living in institutions. *OPCS Surveys of Psychiatric Morbidity in Great Britain*. London: The Stationery Office.

Meltzer, H., Gill, B., Petticrew, M., & Hinds, K. (1996b). Report No. 5, Physical complaints, service use and treatment of residents with psychiatric disorders. *OPCS Surveys of Psychiatric Morbidity in Great Britain*. London: The Stationery Office.

Meltzer, H., Gill, B., Petticrew, M., & Hinds, K. (1996c). Report No. 6, Economic activity and social functioning of residents with psychiatric disorders. *OPCS Surveys of Psychiatric Morbidity in Great Britain*. London: The Stationery Office.

Meltzer, H., Jenkins, R., Singleton, N., Charlton, J., & Yar, M. (1999). *Non-fatal Suicidal Behaviour Among Prisoners*. London: Office for National Statistics.

Menon, D.K. & Peshawaria, R. (2001). Mental retardation in India. In R.S. Murthy (Ed.), *Mental Health in India 1950–2000*. Bangalore: People's Action for Mental Health, pp. 125–138.

Mental Health Europe (1999). *Mental Health Promotion for Children up to 6 Years*. Brussels (www.mhe-sme.org/enmhp)

Mental Health Foundation (2000). *Strategies for Living: Report of User Led Research into People's Strategies for Living with Mental Distress*. London: Mental Health Foundation.

Meyer, M.W. & Zucker, L.G. (1980). *Permanently Failing Organisations.* Newbury Park, CA: Sage.

Miller, N.S. & Swift, R.M. (1997). Primary care medicine and psychiatry: Addictions treatment. *Psychiatric Annals, 27,* 408–416.

Ministry of Health (1998). *Draft Mental Health Act for Zanzibar.* Zanzibar: Ministry of Health.

Mohit, A. (1998). Training packages in developing countries. In R. Jenkins and T.B. Üstün *Preventing Mental Illness –Mental Health Promotion in Primary Care.* Chichester: Wiley.

Morris, J.A. (1995). Alcohol and other drug dependency treatment: A proposal for integration with primary care. *Alcoholism Treatment Quarterly, 13,* 45–57.

Mrazek, P.J. & Haggerty, R.J. (1994). *Reducing the Risks for Mental Disorders: Frontiers for Preventive Intervention Research* Washington, DC: National Academy Press.

Mubbashar, M.H. (2001). Developments in mental health services in Pakistan. In R.S. Murthy (Ed.), *Mental Health in India,* pp. 252–260.

Mubbashar, M.H., Malik, S.J., Zar, J.R., & Wig, N.N. (1986). Community based rural mental health care programme – report of an experiment in Pakistan and Indonesia, involving population groups of 30,000–417,000. *Eastern Mediterranean Health Services Journal,* 14–20.

Mumford, D.B., Saeed, K., Ahmad, I., Latif, S., & Mubbashar, M. (1997). Stress and psychiatric disorder in rural Punjab. A community survey. *British Journal of Psychiatry, 170,* 473–478.

Murray, C.J.L. (1994). Quantifying the burden of disease: The technical basis for disability adjusted life years. *Bulletin of the World Health Organisation, 72,* 429–445.

Murray, C.J.L., Lopez, A.D., & Jamison, D.T. (1994). The global burden of disease in 1990: Summary results, sensitivity analysis and future directions. *Bulletin of the World Health Organisation, 72(3),* 495–509.

Murray, C.J.L. & Lopez, A.D. (1996). *The Global Burden of Disease – A comprehensive assessment of mortality and disability from diseases, injuries and risk factors in 1990 and projected to 2020.* Boston: Harvard University Press.

Murray, C.J.L. & Lopez, A.D. (1999). *Global Burden of Disease.* World Health Organization.

Murray, J. & Jenkins, R. (1998). Prevention of mental illness in primary care. *International Review of Psychiatry, 10,* 154–157.

Murthy, R. (1983). Treatment and rehabilitation of the severely mentally ill in developing countries. Experience of countries in South East Asia. *International Journal of Mental Health, 12,* 16–29.

Murthy, R. (1997). Application of intervention in developing countries. In R. Jenkins & T.B. Ustun (Eds), *Preventing Mental Illness: Mental Health Promotion in Developing Countries.* Chichester: Wiley.

Murthy, R. & Burns, B. (Eds), (1992). *Community Mental Health Proceedings of Indo–US Symposium.* Bangalore: National Institute of Mental Health and Neuroscience.

Murthy, S. & Wig, N. (1983). A training approach to enhancing mental health manpower in a developing country. *American Journal of Psychiatry, 140,* 1486–1490.

Naik, U.S. (2001). Child Psychiatry in India – the last quarter century. In R.S. Murthy (Ed.), *Mental Health in India 1950–2000.* pp. 108–124.

Nicholson, D.W. (1995). The future of psychology in a changing health care marketplace: A conversation with Russ Newman. *Professional Psychology Research and Practice, 26,* 366–370.

Neki, J.S., Joinet, B., Ndosi, N., Kilonzo, G., Hauli, J.G., & Duvinage, G. (1986). Witchcraft and psychotherapy. *British Journal of Psychiatry, 149,* 145–155.

Niedhammer, I. & Goldberg, M. (1998). Psychosocial work environment and cardiovascular risk factors in an occupational cohort in France. *Journal of Epidemiology and Community Health*, *52*, 93–100.

North, F., Smye, S.L., Freeney, A., Head, J., Shipley, M.J., & Marmot, M.G. (1993). Explaining socio-economic differences in sickness absence: The Whitehall II study. *British Medical Journal*, *306*, 361–365.

O'Dea, J. & Abraham, S. (1999). Improving the body image, eating attitudes and behaviours of young male and female adolescents: A new educational approach which focuses on self-esteem. *Journal of Abnormal Psychology*, *99*, 3–15.

Odejide, A.O., Ogunleya, D.A., & Meletoyitan, F.S. (1993). *Pattern of psychoactive drug use/abuse in northern Nigeria secondary schools: The Kano City example.* Paper presented at CRISA 2nd Biennial Conference in Jos, Plateau State, Nigeria, 24–25 June.

Office for National Statistics (1998). *Labour Force Survey 1997/8.* London: Office for National Statistics.

Ojamunga, D.N. (1981). What doctors think of traditional healers and vice versa. *World Health Forum*, *2*, 407–410.

Olds, D.L. (1998). The prenatal/early infancy project. In R.H. Price et al. (Eds), *14 Ounces of Prevention: A Casebook for Practitioners.* Washington: American Psychological Association.

Olds, D.L., Eckenrode, J., Henderson, C.R., Kitzman, H., Powers, J., Cole, R., Sidora, K., Morris, P., Pettitt, L.M., & Luckey, D. (1997). Long term effects of home visitation on maternal life course and child abuse and neglect: Fifteen year follow up of a randomised trial. *Journal of American Medical Association*, *278*, 637–643.

Olweus, D. (1993). *Bullying at School: What we Know and What we can Do.* London: Blackwell.

Onyett, S., Piollenger, T., & Muijen, M. (1996). *Making Community Mental Health Teams Work: CMHTs and the people who work in them.* London: Sainsbury Centre for Mental Health.

Ormel, J., Von Korff, M., Ustun, T., Pini, S., Korten, A., & Oldehinkel, T. (1994). Common mental disorders and disability across cultures: Results from the WHO Collaborative study on psychological problems in primary care. *Journal of American Medical Association*, *272*, 1741–1748.

Pai, S. & Kapur, R.L. (1983). Evaluation of home care treatment for schizophrenic patients. *Acta Psychiatrica Scandinavica*, *67*, 18–88.

Pan-American Health Organisation (1981). *Emergency Health Management After Natural Disasters.* Scientific Publication No 407. Washington DC: Pan-American Health Organisation.

Parker, C. & McCulloch, A.W. (1999). *Key Issues from Homicide Inquiries.* London: Mind.

Parry, C.D.H. (1996). A review of psychiatric epidemiology in Africa: Strategies for increasing validity when using instruments transculturally. *Transcultural Psychiatric Research Review*, *33*, 173–188.

Patel, V. (2000). The epidemiology of common mental disorders in South Asia. *NIMHANS Journal* – special issue on the Epidemiology of Neurological and Psychiatric Disorders in India (in press).

Patel, V., Gwanzura, F., Simunyu, E., Mann, A., & Lloyd, K. (1995). The explanatory models and phenomenology of common mental disorders in Harare, Zimbabwe. *Psychological Medicine*, *25*, 1191–1199.

Patel, V., Pereira, J., Coutunho, L., & Fernadez, R. (1998). Poverty, psychological disorder and disability in primary care attenders in Goa, India. *British Journal of Psychiatry*, *172*, 533–536.

Patterson, M.G., West, M.A., Lawthorn, R., & Nickell, S. (1997). *Impact of People Management Practices on Business Performance*. Institute for Personnel and Development.

Paykel, E.S., Abbott, R., Jenkins, R., Brugha, T.S., & Meltzer, H. (2000). Urban–rural mental health differences in Great Britain: Findings from the National Morbidity Survey. *Psychological Medicine, 30*, 269–280.

Peersman, G., Harden, A., & Oliver, S. (1998). *Effectiveness of Health Promotion Interventions in the Workplace: A Review*. London: Health Education Authority.

Peters, J., Brooker, C., McCabe, C., & Short, N. (1998). Problems encountered with opportunistic screening for alcohol related problems in patients attending an A&E department. *Addiction, 93*, 589–594.

Pfeffer, J. (1998). *The Human Equation: Building Profits by Putting People First*. Harvard Business School Press: Cambridge, USA.

Philips, R. & Robertson, I. (1996). Poetry helps healing. *Lancet, 347*, 332–333.

Phillips, M., Liu, H., & Zhang, Y. (1999). Suicide and social change in China. *Cultural and Medical Psychiatry, 23*, 5–50.

Philo, G. (1996). *Media and Mental Distress*. London: Addison Wesley Longman.

Pollack, D. & Goetz, R. (1997). Psychiatric interface with primary care. In K. Minkoff & D. Pollack (Eds), *Managed Mental Health Care in the Public Sector: A Survival Manual*. Amsterdam: Harwood.

Pollin, I. & DeLeon, P.H. (1996). Integrated health delivery systems: Psychology's potential role. *Professional Psychology Research and Practice, 27*, 107–108.

Pransky, J. (1991). *Prevention: The Critical Need*. Springfield, MO: Burrely Foundation and Paradigm Press.

Price, R.H. (1998). Theoretical frameworks for mental health risk reduction in primary care. In R. Jenkins & T.B. Ustun (Eds), *Preventing Mental Illness: Mental Health Promotion in Primary Care*. Chichester: Wiley.

Price, R.H., Van Ryn, M., & Vinokur, A.D. (1992). Impact of a preventive job search intervention on the likelihood of depression among the unemployed. *Journal of Health and Social Behaviour, 33*. 158–167.

Pucheu, R.C. (1985). Attencion primaria y fomento a la salud mental. *Cuestion Social, 2*, 74–82.

Putnam, R.D. (1995). Bowling alone: America's declining social capital. *Journal of Democracy, 6*, 65–78.

Rahman, A., Mubbashar, M., Gater, R., & Goldberg, D. (1998). Randomised trial of impact of school mental health programme in rural Rawalpindi, Pakistan. *Lancet, 352*, 1022–1025.

Rainford, L., Mason, V., Hickman, M., & Morgan, A. (2000). *Health in England 1998: Investigating the Links between Social Inequalities and Health*. London: The Stationery Office.

Rane, A.J. (2000). Hamara Club: A project for street children. *The Indian Journal of Social Work, 61* (Issue 2).

Regier, D.A., Goldberg, I.D., & Taube. C.A. (1978). The 'de facto' US mental health service systems. *Archives of General Psychiatry, 35*, 685–693..

Reich, M.R. (1993). The political economy of health transitions in the third world. In L.C. Chen, A. Kleinman & N.C. Ware (Eds), *Health and Social Change in International Perspectives*, pp. 411–451. Cambridge, MA: Harvard University Press.

Repper, J., Sayce, L., Strong, S., Willmot, J., & Haines, M. (1997). *Tall Stories from the Back Yard. A Survey of 'nimby' opposition to community mental health facilities, experienced by key service providers in England and Wales*. London: Mind Publications.

Richeport, M. (1984). Strategies and outcomes of introducing a mental health plan in Brazil. *Social Science and Medicine, 19*, 261–271.

Richter, L.M. (1994). Any kinds of deprivation: Young children and their families. In *South Africa in Early Intervention and Culture: Preparation for Literacy: The Interface between Theory and Practice*. UNESCO, pp. 95–113.

Rick, J., Perryman, S., Young, K., Guppy, A., & Hillage, J. (1998). *Workplace trauma and its management. A review of the literature*. The Institute for Employment Studies, Suffolk. Published by HSE Books.

Robson, M.H., France, R., & Bland, M. (1984). Clinical psychologist in primary care controlled clinical and economic evaluation. *British Medical Journal, 288*, 1805–1808.

Rose, D. (1996). *Living in the Community*. London: Sainsbury Centre for Mental Health.

Rosengren, A., et al. (1993). Stressful life events, social supports and morbidity in men born in 1933. *British Medical Journal, 307*, 1102–1105.

Rosenthal, E. & Rubenstein, S. (1993). International Human Rights Advocacy under the 'Principles for the Protection of Persons with Mental Illness'. *International Journal of Law and Psychiatry, 16*, pp. 257–300.

Rubenstein, L.V., Lammers, J., Yano, E.M., Tabbarah, M., & Robbins, A.S, (1996). Evaluation of the VA's pilot programme in institutional reorganization toward primary and ambulatory: Part II, a study of organizational stresses and dynamics. *Academic Medicine, 71*, 784–792.

Rutter, M. (1985). Resilience in the face of adversity: Protective factors and resistance to psychiatric disorder. *British Journal of Psychiatry, 147*, 598–611.

Rutter, M. & Smith, D.J. (1995). *Psychosocial Disorders in Young People*. Chichester: Wiley.

Rutter, M. & Quinton, D. (1984). Parental psychiatric disorder: Effects on children. *Psychological Medicine, 14*, 853–880.

Rutz, W., von Knorring, L., & Walinder, J. (1989). Frequency of suicide on Gotland after systematic postgraduate education of general practitioners. *Acta Psychiatrica Scandinavica, 80*, 151–154.

Rutz, W., von Knorring, L., Walinder, J. & Wistedt, B. (1990). Effect of an educational programme for general practitioners on Gotland on the pattern of prescription of psychotropic drugs. *Acta Psychiatrica Scandinavica, 82*, 399–403.

Rutz, W., von Knorring, L., Philgren, H. & Rihmer, Z. (1995). Prevention of male suicides: Lessons from the Gotland study. *Lancet, 345*, 524.

Saeed, K., Wtrz, S., Gater, R., Mubbashar, M.H., Tomkins, A., & Sullivan, K. (1999). Detection of disabilities by school children – a pilot study in rural Pakistan. *Tropical Doctor, 29*, 151–155.

Saeed, K., Gater, R., Mubbashar, M.H., & Hussain, A. (2000). The prevalence, classification and treatment of mental disorders among attendees of native healers in rural Pakistan. *Journal of Social Psychiatry and Psychiatric Epidemiology, 35*, 480–485.

Salon, R. & Maretzki, T. (1983). Mental health services and traditional healing in Indonesia – are the roles compatible? *Culture, Medicine and Psychiatry, 7*, 277–412.

Sartorius, N. (1990). Mental health care in continental Europe: Medley or mosaic? In I.M. Marks & R.A. Scott (Eds), *Mental Health Care Delivery: Innovations, Impediments and Implementation*, pp. 154–155. New York: Sage.

Sartorius, N. & Harding, T. (1983). The WHO collaborative study on strategies for extending mental health care/The genesis of the study. *American Journal of Psychiatry, 140*, 1470–1479.

Saxena, S. (2001). Alcohol related problems in India. In R. Murthy (Ed.), *Mental Health in India – Essays in honour of Professor Wig 1950–2000*. Bangalore: People's Action for Mental Health.

Sayce, L. & Morris, D. (1999). *Outsiders Coming In? Achieving Social Inclusion for People with Mental Health Problems*. London: Mind Publications.

Schweinhart, L.J. & Weikart, D.P. (1992). High/Scope Perry Preschool Program outcomes. in J. McCord & R.E.D. Tremblay (Eds), *Preventing Anti-social Behaviour: Interventions from Birth through Adolescence*. New York: Guilford Press, pp. 67–86.

Schulsinger, F. & Jablensky, A. (1991). The national mental health programme in the United Republic of Tanzania: A report from WHO and DANIDA. *Acta Psychiatrica Scandinavica, 83*, 132.

SCMH (1998). *Keys to Engagement*. London: Sainsbury Centre for Mental Health.

SCMH (2000). *Finding and Keeping: Review of Recruitment and Retention in the Mental Health Workforce*. London: Sainsbury Centre for Mental Health.

Scott, K.D., Klaus, P.H., & Klaus, M.H. (1999). The obstetrical and postpartum benefits of continuous support during childbirth. *Journal of Women's Health and Gender Based Medicine, 8*, 1257–1264.

Seboron, G., Frank, J. & Sepulveda, J. (1986). The health care reform in Mexico – Before and after the 1985 earthquake. *American Journal of Public Health, 76*, 673–680 (and for integrating mental health care into general health services).

Shah, A. & Jenkins, R. (2000). Mental health economic studies from developing countries reviewed in the context of those from developed countries. *Acta Psychiatrica Scandinavica, 101*, 87–103.

Shapiro, J. & Talbot, Y. (1992). Is there a future for behavioural scientists in academic family medicine. *Family Systems Medicine, 10*, 247–256.

Shah, A., Jenkins, R. & Saraceno, B. (2000). Nations for mental health and old age psychiatry. *International Psychiatric Association Bulletin*, 19–20.

Shepherd, M., Cooper, B., Brown, A.C., Katon, G. et al. (1966). *Psychiatric Illness in General Practice*. London: Oxford University Press.

Shepherd, M. (1980). Mental health as an integrant of primary medical care. *Journal of the Royal College of General Practitioners, 30*, 657–664.

Simon, G.E., Van Korff, M., Piccinelli, M., Fullerton, C., & Ormel, P. (1999). An international study of the relations between somatic symptoms and depression. *New England Journal of Medicine, 341*, 1329–1334.

Singleton, N., Meltzer, H., & Gatward, R., with Coid, J. & Deasy, D. (1998). *Psychiatric Morbidity among Prisoners in England and Wales*. London: Office for National Statistics.

Smith, R. (1981). Alcohol, women and the young: The same old problem. *British Medical Journal, 288*, 308–310.

Smith, A.P., Wadsworth, E. et al. (2000). *The Scale of Occupational Stress: The Bristol Stress and Health at Work Study*. London: Health and Safety Executive.

Social Exclusion Unit (2000). *National Strategy for Neighbourhood Renewal: A Framework for Consultation*. Cabinet Office.

Spector, R.E. (1979). *Cultural Diversity in Health and Illness*. USA: LCC Publishers.

Stansfield, S., Head, J. & Marmot, M. (2000). *Work-related factors and ill health: The Whitehall II study*. Suffolk: HSE.

Stark, W. (1998). Empowerment and self-help initiatives – enhancing the quality of psychosocial care. In R. Jenkins & T.B. Ustun (Eds), *Preventing Mental Illness: Mental Health Promotion in Primary Care*, pp. 291–297.

Stein, L. & Test, M.A. (1980). Alternatives to mental hospital treatment. *Archives of General Psychiatry, 37*, 392–397.

Stewart-Brown, S. (1998). Emotional well-being and its relation to health. *British Medical Journal, 317*, 1608–1609.

Strathdee, G. & Jenkins, R. (1996). Purchasing mental health care for primary care. In G. Thornicroft & G. Strathdee (Eds). *Commissioning Mental Health Services*. London: HMSO, pp. 71–83.

Strathdee, G. & Thornicroft, G. (1996). Core components of a comprehensive mental health service. In G. Thornicroft & G. Strathdee (Eds), *Commissioning Mental Health Services*. London: HMSO, pp. 133–145.

Strathdee, G. & Williams, P. (1984). A survey of psychiatrists in primary care: The silent growth of a new service. *Journal of the Royal College of Practitioners*, *34*, 615–618.

Summerfield, D. (2000). War and mental health: A brief overview. *British Medical Journal*, *320*, 232–235.

Swantz, M.L. (1990). *The Medicine Man among the Zaramo of Dar-es-Salaam* (ed. Mai Palmberg). The Scandinavian Institute of African Studies and the University of Dar-es-Salaam Press.

Swantz, M.L. (1979). Community and healing among the Zaramo in Tanzania. *Social Science and Medicine*, *138*, 169–173.

Szmuckler, G.I. (1985). The epidemiology of anorexia nervosa and bulimia. *British Journal of Psychiatric Research*, *19*, 143–153.

Tadmor, C.S. (1988). The perceived personal control preventive intervention for a caesarean birth population. In R.H. Price et al. (Eds), *Fourteen Ounces of Prevention: A Casebook for Practitioners*, pp. 141–152. Washington, DC: American Psychological Association.

Tadmor, C.S., Bas-Maor, J.A., Birkhan, J., Shoshany, G., & Hofman, J.E. (1998). Paediatric surgery: A preventive intervention approach to the mastery of stress. *Journal of Preventive Psychiatry*, *3*, 4.

Tarnopolsky, A. & Clark, C. (1984). Environmental noise and mental health. In H.L. Freeman (Ed). *Mental Health and the Environment*, pp. 250–270.

Tausig, M. & Subedi, S. (1997). The Modern Mental Health System in Nepal: Organisational persistence in the absence of legitimatising myths. *Social Science and Medicine*, *45*, 441–447.

Taylor, P.J. & Gunn, J. (1999). Homicides by people with mental illness: Myth and reality. *British Journal of Psychiatry*, *174*, 9–14.

Taylor, S.J., Kingdon, D., & Jenkins, R. (1997). How are nations trying to prevent suicide? An analysis of national suicide prevention strategies. *Acta Psychiatrica Scandinavica*, *95*, 457–463.

Thompson, C. (1989). *The Instruments of Psychiatric Research*. Chichester: Wiley.

Thornicroft, G. & Strathdee, G. (Eds), (1996). *Commissioning Mental Health Services*. London: HMSO.

Tomlinson, D. & Carrier, J. (1996). *Asylum in the Community*. London: Routledge.

Turner, J. & Kelly, B. (2000). Emotional dimensions of chronic disease. *British Medical Journal*, *172*, 124–128.

UNICEF (1999). The State of the World's Children – Education. New York: UNICEF.

United Nations (1996). *Prevention of Suicide Guidelines for the Formulation and Implementation of National Strategies*. New York: United Nations.

Ustun, T.B. & Sartorius, N. (1995). *Mental Illness in General Health Care – An International Study*. Chichester: Wiley.

Vargas, R. (1979). Health policies in Latin America. *Social Science and Medicine*, *13C*, 72.

Vazquez-Barquero, J., Munoz, P., & Madoz Jawegi, V. (1981). The interaction between physical illness and neurotic morbidity in the community. *British Journal of Psychiatry*, *139*, 328–333.

Vazquez-Barquero, J., Pena, C., Diez Manrique, J.F., & Lianoa Rincon, A. (1991). Risk profiles for mental disorders in the general population. *Actas Luso Esp Neurol Psiquitari Cieric Afines*, *19*, 62–76.

Vedhara, K., Cox, N.K., & Wilcock, G.K. (1999). Chronic stress in elderly carers of dementia patients and antibody response to influenza vaccination. *Lancet*, *353*, 627–631.

Villeneau, L., Morris, D., Parkman, S., Wolf, J. & McCulloch, A. (2000). *On Your Doorstep: Community Organisations and Mental Health*. London: Sainsbury Centre for Mental Health.

Vinokur, A.D. & Ryn, V. (1991). Long term follow up and benefit cost analysis of the JOBS program: A preventive intervention for the unemployed. *Journal of Applied Psychology, 76*, 213–219.

Vinokur, A.D., Price, R.H., & Schul, Y. (1995). Impact of the JOBS intervention on unemployed workers varying in risk for depression. *American Journal of Community Psychology, 23*, 39–74.

Wallcraft, J. (1998). *Healing Minds: A report on current research, policy and practice concerning the use of complementary and alternative therapies for a wide range of mental health problems*. London: The Mental Health Foundation.

Ward, E., King, M., Lloyd, M., Bower, P., Shibbald, B., Farrelly, S., Gabbay, M., Tarrier, N. & Addington-Hall, J. (2000). Randomised controlled trail of non-directive counselling, cognitive behaviour therapy and usual general practitioner care for patients with depression: Clinical effectiveness. *British Medical Journal, 321*, 1383–1388.

Watt, I.S., Franks, A.J., & Sheldon, T.A. (1994). Health and health care of rural populations in the UK: Is it better or worse? *Journal of Epidemiology and Community Health, 48*, 16–21.

Weare, K. & Gray, G. (1995). Promoting mental and emotional health. In *The European Network of Health Promoting Schools*. WHO/Council of Europe.

Weiss, M. (1985). The inter-relationship of tropical disease and mental disorder: Conceptual framework and literature review. *Culture, Medicine and Psychiatry, 9*, 121–200.

Weissman, M., Myers, J., & Harding, P. (1978). Psychiatric disorders in a US urban community: 1975–76. *American Journal of Psychiatry, 135*, 459–466.

Wessely, S., Rose, S., & Bisson, J. (1999). *A systematic review of brief psychological interventions 'debriefing' for the treatment of immediate trauma-related symptoms and the prevention of post traumatic stress disorder*. Cochrane Collaboration, Cochrane Library, Issue 4. Oxford: Update Software.

Wheeler, F.A., Gore, K.M., & Greenblatt, B. (1998). The beneficial effects of volunteering for older volunteers and the people they serve: A meta analysis. *International Journal of Ageing and Human Development, 47*, 69–79.

Whelan, C.T. (1993). The role of social support in mediating the psychological consequences of economic stress. *Sociology of Health and Illness, 15*, 86–101.

White, E. (1990). *The Third Quinquennial National CPN Survey*. Manchester: Department of Nursing, University of Manchester.

WHO (1975). *Recommendation 10: Organisation of Mental Health Services in Developing Countries*. Technical Report Series 812. Geneva: World Health Organisation.

WHO (1978). *Report and Declaration from the World Health Organisation*, Alma Ata, USSR. Geneva: World Health Organisation.

WHO (1979). *Report of the International Conference on Primary Health Care*, Alma Ata, USSR. Geneva: World Health Organisation.

WHO (1984). *Mental Health Care in Developing Countries. Report of a WHO Study Group*. Technical Report Series 698. Geneva: World Health Organisation.

WHO (1991). *Guidelines for the Assessment of Herbal Medicines*. Geneva: World Health Organisation.

WHO (1992). *Twenty Steps for Developing a Healthy Cities Project*. Copenhagen: World Health Regional Office for Europe.

WHO (1993). *The ICD-10 Classification of Mental and Behavioural Disorders – Diagnostic Criteria for Research*. Geneva: World Health Organisation.

WHO (1996b). *Mental Health of Refugees*. Geneva: World Health Organisation.

WHO (2000). *Health in Emergencies: The Experience in the Former Yugoslav Republic of Macedonia in 1999*. Report from the workshop, Skopje, May 2000. WHO Regional office for Europe, Humanitarian assistance Office, Skopje, FYR Macedonia.

WHO Collaborating Centre (2000). *WHO Guide to Mental Health in Primary Care* (adapted for the UK from *Diagnostic and Management Guidelines for Mental Disorders in Primary Care*, Chapter V, *Primary Care Version*. London: Royal Society of Medicine.

WHO Collaborating Centre (2002). *Guide to Mental Health in Prisons* (adapted for the UK from *Diagnostic and Management Guidelines for Mental Disorders in Primary Care*). Chapter V, Primary Care version). London: Royal Society Medicine.

Wig, N. & Murthy, S. (1994). From mental illness to mental health. *Health for the Millions*, *20*, 2–4.

Wilkinson, R. (2000). Inequality and the social environment: A reply to Lynch et al. *Journal of Epidemiological Community Health*, *54*, 411–413.

Williams, S., Michie, S., & Pattani, S. (1998). *Improving the Health of the NHS Workforce*. Report of the partnership on the health of the NHS Workforce. Leeds: The Nuffield Trust.

Wing, J.K. (1992). *Epidemiologically based Needs Assessment: Mental Illness*. London: NHSME.

Wing, J.K., Curtis, R.H., & Beevor, A.S. (1996). *HoNOS: The Health of the Nation Outcome Scales. Report on Research and Development 1993–1995*. London: Royal College of Psychiatrists.

Wolf, G., Pathare, S., Craig, T. et al. (1999). Public education for community care: A new approach. In J. Guimon, W. Fischer & N. Sartorius (Eds), *The Image of Madness: The Public facing Mental Illness and Psychiatric Treatment*, pp. 105–117. Basel: Karger.

Wood, H. & Carr, S. (1998). *Locality Services in Mental Health: Developing Home Treatment and Assertive Outreach*. London: The Sainsbury Centre for Mental Health/ North Birmingham Mental Health NHS Trust.

Wootton, B. (1959). *Social Science and Social Pathology*, Chapter 7, pp. 203–226. London: George Allen and Unwin.

World Bank (1993). *Investing in Health*. World Development Report 1993. Washington, DC: World Bank.

World Medical Association (1964). *World Medical Association Declaration of Helsinki*. Adopted by the 18th World Medical Assembly, Helsinki, Finland, June 1964. http://ohsr.od.nih.gov/helsinki.php3

Wynne-Owen, J. (1998). The declaration of Windsor. *Arts, Health and Well-being: Beyond the Millennium. the Role of Humanities in Medicine*. London: The Nuffield Trust.

Yamey, G. (2000). Psychologists question 'debriefing' for traumatised employees. *British Medical Journal*, *320*, 140.

Yule, W. & Canterbury, R. (1994). The treatment of post traumatic stress disorder in children and adolescents. *International Review of Psychiatry*, *6*, 141–151.

Zeichner, C.I. (1988). *Modern and Traditional Health Care in Developing Societies*. Lanham, MD: University Press of America.

Zoritch. B., Roberts, I., & Oakley. A. (2000). Daycare for pre-school children. *Cochrane Review, The Cochrane Library*, Issue 3. Oxford: Update Software.

Author index

Subject index

Printed in Great Britain
by Amazon